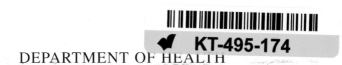
DEPARTMENT OF HEALTH

On the State of
THE PUBLIC HEALTH

THE ANNUAL REPORT OF
THE CHIEF MEDICAL OFFICER OF
THE DEPARTMENT OF HEALTH
FOR THE YEAR 1993

LONDON
HMSO

CONTENTS

INTRODUCTION   1

EXECUTIVE SUMMARY   7

1. VITAL STATISTICS   29
    (a) Population size   29
    (b) Age and sex structure of the resident population   29
    (c) Fertility statistics - aspects of relevance for health care 29
    (d) Mortality   35
    (e) Prevalence of disease in the community   38
    (f) Infant and perinatal mortality   42
    (g) Trends in cancer incidence and mortality   43
    (h) Trends in reporting congenital malformations   44
    (i) Appendix Tables and their content (pages 203-213)   44

2. THE NATION'S HEALTH   46
    (a) Public health in England   46
    (b) Regional perspectives   48
    (c) Inter-Departmental Group on Public Health   52
    (d) Sickness at work   52
    (e) Urban health   53
    (f) Variations in health   54
    (g) Health of people in later life   55
    (h) Health of black and ethnic minorities   56
    (i) Health of men   57

3. THE STRATEGY FOR HEALTH   60
    (a) One year on   60
    (b) Key areas and targets   61
         (i)   Coronary heart disease and stroke   61
         (ii)   Cancers   63
         (iii) Mental illness   65
         (iv)   HIV/AIDS and sexual health   66
         (v)   Accidents   67
    (c) Nutrition   69
    (d) Implementation   70
         (i)   NHS activities   70
         (ii)   Local health alliances   71
         (iii) Healthy settings   71
         (iv)   Inter-Departmental co-operation   72
    (e) The way ahead   73

4. THE HEALTH OF ADOLESCENTS   74
    (a) Mortality   77
    (b) Morbidity   80
    (c) Specific conditions   89
         (i)   Injury   89
         (ii)   Cancer   89
         (iii) Diabetes mellitus   89
         (iv)   Asthma   89
         (v)   Sexually transmitted diseases   91

	(vi)	Dental health	94
(d)		Lifestyle and health	95
	(i)	Physical activity	96
	(ii)	Diet and nutrition	96
	(iii)	Smoking	96
	(iv)	Alcohol misuse	96
	(v)	Substance misuse	97
	(vi)	Sexual behaviour	97
	(vii)	Mental health	99
(e)		Social factors	102
	(i)	Child protection	102
	(ii)	Children looked after by Local Authorities	102
	(iii)	Divorce	105
	(iv)	Violence	105
	(v)	Unauthorised school absence	107
	(vi)	Employment	107
	(vii)	Homelessness	107
(f)		Health services for adolescents	110
(g)		Improving the health of adolescents	111

5. HEALTH CARE — 113

(a)		Needs, effectiveness and outcomes	113
	(i)	Health needs assessment	113
	(ii)	Basic sources of information	113
	(iii)	National confidential enquiries	115
	(iv)	Quality of service and effectiveness of care	115
	(v)	Clinical standards and guidelines	116
	(vi)	Clinical audit in primary care	116
	(vii)	Health outcomes	117
(b)		Primary health care	119
	(i)	Organisation of primary care	119
	(ii)	Prescribing	120
	(iii)	Professional development and clinical audit	121
	(iv)	The way ahead	121
(c)		Hospital services	122
	(i)	Specialised services	122
	(ii)	Cancer	122
	(iii)	National Confidential Enquiry into Peri-operative Deaths	123
(d)		Diabetes mellitus	123
(e)		Asthma	124
(f)		Osteopathy and chiropractic	125
(g)		Mental health	126
	(i)	Mental health and primary care	126
	(ii)	Occupational mental health	126
	(iii)	Services for people with severe mental illness	127
	(iv)	Services for mentally disordered offenders	127
	(v)	Mental health legislation	129
(h)		Maternity and child health services	130
	(i)	Report of the Expert Maternity Group	130
	(ii)	Confidential Enquiries into Maternal Deaths	131
	(iii)	Folic acid and neural tube defects	131
	(iv)	Vitamin A and pregnancy	131
	(v)	Human Fertilisation and Embryology Authority	131

		(vi)	Sudden infant death syndrome	132
		(vii)	Prophylaxis of vitamin K deficiency bleeding in infants	132
		(viii)	Neonatal intensive care	133
		(ix)	Paediatric intensive care	134
		(x)	Confidential Enquiry into Stillbirths and Deaths in Infancy	134
		(xi)	Notification of congenital malformations	135
		(xii)	Gene Therapy Advisory Committee	136
	(i)	Learning disabilities		137
	(j)	Disability and rehabilitation		138
	(k)	Prison health care		139

6.	COMMUNICABLE DISEASES		141
	(a)	HIV infection and AIDS	141
	(b)	Other sexually transmitted diseases	151
	(c)	Immunisation	154
	(d)	Hepatitis B guidelines	156
	(e)	Influenza	156
	(f)	Tuberculosis	157
	(g)	Foodborne and waterborne diseases	158
	(h)	Travel-related disease	162

7.	ENVIRONMENTAL HEALTH AND TOXICOLOGY		164
	(a)	Chemical and physical agents in the environment		164
		(i)	Small Area Health Statistics Unit	164
		(ii)	Air pollution episodes	164
		(iii)	Institute for Environment and Health	165
		(iv)	NHS response to chemical accidents	166
		(v)	Distribution of stable iodine	166
	(b)	Toxicological safety		167
		(i)	Food chemical hazards	167
		(ii)	Food carcinogen prioritisation	167
		(iii)	Mineral hydrocarbons in food	168
		(iv)	The Advisory Committee on Novel Foods and Processes	168
		(v)	Pesticides	168
		(vi)	Veterinary drugs and animal feedingstuffs	168
		(vii)	Sheep dips	169

8.	MEDICAL EDUCATION, TRAINING AND STAFFING		171
	(a)	Junior doctors' hours	171
	(b)	'Achieving a Balance'	171
	(c)	Medical Manpower Standing Advisory Committee	172
	(d)	Equal opportunities for doctors	172
	(e)	Part-time consultant scheme	173
	(f)	New career structure for doctors in community health	174
	(g)	Postgraduate, continuing and specialist medical education	174
	(h)	Undergraduate medical and dental education	175
	(i)	Doctors' performance	176
	(j)	Locum doctors	176

9.	OTHER TOPICS OF INTEREST IN 1993		177
	(a)	Medicines Control Agency		177
		(i)	Role and performance	177
		(ii)	Control of UK clinical trials	177

	(iii)	Reclassification of medicines from Prescription Only to Pharmacy status	178
	(iv)	Control of gene therapy products	178
	(v)	Other pharmaceutical developments in the European Community	179
(b)		The European Medicines Evaluation Agency and pharmaceutical licensing systems	179
(c)		National Blood Authority	180
(d)		Creutzfeldt-Jakob disease surveillance	180
(e)		Medical devices	182
(f)		Bioethics	184
	(i)	Local Research Ethics Committees	184
	(ii)	Bioethics in Europe	184
	(iii)	Committee on the Ethics of Gene Therapy	185
	(iv)	Ethics of genetic screening	186
	(v)	Lifestyle and treatment	186
(g)		London Implementation Group	187
(h)		Research and development	188
	(i)	Report of the Advisory Council on Science and Technology	188
	(ii)	White Paper on science, engineering and technology	189
	(iii)	Research for health	189
(i)		Dental health	190
	(i)	Dental health of the nation	190
	(ii)	General dental services	190
	(iii)	Community dental services	191
	(iv)	Hospital dental services	192
	(v)	Continuing education and training for dentists	192
	(vi)	Dental research	193

10.	INTERNATIONAL HEALTH		194
(a)		England, Europe and health	194
(b)		The European Community	194
	(i)	Treaty on European Union (Maastricht)	194
	(ii)	European Economic Area	195
	(iii)	The Council of Health Ministers	195
	(iv)	EC/WHO/Council of Europe	195
	(v)	Free movement of people	195
	(vi)	Draft Directive on Data Protection	196
	(vii)	Smoking	196
	(viii)	Elderly and disabled people	196
	(ix)	AIDS and HIV infection	197
	(x)	Pharmaceuticals	197
	(xi)	Research and information technology	197
	(xii)	Food safety	198
(c)		Relations with Central and Eastern Europe	198
(d)		Council of Europe	200
(e)		The Commonwealth	200
(f)		WHO	201
	(i)	European Regional Committee	201
	(ii)	Executive Board	201
	(iii)	World Health Assembly	202

APPENDIX	203

INTRODUCTION

Rt Hon Virginia Bottomley MP
Secretary of State for Health

Madam,

I have pleasure in submitting my Report on the State of the Public Health for 1993, together with some comments on the more important developments and events in the first half of 1994. This Report is the 136th of the series which began in 1858.

I am pleased to report that there were considerable improvements in health over the year: introduction of *Haemophilus influenzae* type b vaccine has already had a significant impact on reported infections, and the White Paper *The Health of the Nation: a strategy for health in England*[1] continues to provide an important impetus for improving health. Launched in July 1992, it has been taken up with vigour by a wide range of organisations, including the voluntary sector. For most of the targets set, progress is in the right direction although, as is pointed out in this Report, some targets present particular challenges.

As I discussed last year, this Report is not simply a document of record, but must also try to interpret and to explain changes in those factors that are known to influence and to determine health, and should identify areas where improvements could be made. In previous years, I have highlighted some issues for special mention, with the intention that they would be followed up in subsequent Reports. Topics identified in 1991 and 1992 have been acted on and progress is discussed in this Report. Four key issues are identified for broader discussion during the coming year: the health of adolescents, genetic factors and disease, the changing patterns of infectious diseases, and asthma. It is hoped that over the next year these four topics will stimulate interest, and I shall report back on these areas in next year's Report.

I wish to acknowledge the help and support given to me by numerous colleagues in the Department of Health and the Office of Population Censuses and Surveys in the preparation of this Report, and the assistance of Her Majesty's Stationery Office, Norwich, which arranged the printing and publication. I am also grateful to the Regional Directors of Public Health who have contributed to this year's and to last year's Report.

I am, Madam,
Your obedient servant

Kenneth C Calman

September 1994

LONG-TERM STRATEGIC AIMS

Last year's Report[2] set out a series of long-term strategic aims which also underpin the content of this Report:

- To promote efforts to ensure health for all;

- To achieve the targets in the strategy for health;

- To involve patients and the public in choices and decision-making;

- To establish an effective intelligence and information system for public health and clinical practice;

- To ensure a health service based on an assessment of health needs, quality of care and effectiveness of outcome; *and*

- To provide a highly professional team of staff with strong educational, research and ethical standards.

These six points continue to provide the strategic direction and intent of the Report.

HEALTH IN ENGLAND IN 1993

Life expectancy continues to increase and in 1992 the lowest infant mortality rate of 6.5 per 1,000 live births was achieved. Immunisation coverage continues to rise and an increasing number of District Health Authorities (DHAs) are now reaching 95% coverage for all immunisations. The introduction of *Haemophilus influenzae* type b (Hib) vaccination has reduced laboratory reports of meningitis and septicaemia by 85% in children under 1 year-of-age.

The age and sex structure of the population remains fairly stable. It should be noted, however, that there is still a rapid increase in the number of people aged 85 years and over, three-quarters of whom are women; considerable thought must be given to the provision of care and support for the elderly. Over three-quarters of all National Health Service (NHS) patients consult health care professionals in general practice during the course of a year, with the highest proportions seen among children under the age of 5 years, and among adults aged over 65 years.

During 1993, there was an earlier than usual rise in the number of cases of influenza, which resulted in a higher than expected death rate. Prediction of the type of influenza likely to circulate, the production of an appropriate vaccine, and the immunisation of high-risk groups is a cyclical problem, and for the coming year I have already begun to alert the public and health care professionals to this process[3].

Variations in health and health care still exist, and are related to a wide range of factors. Various initiatives were begun early this year to improve our understanding of the issues and to reduce variations. The Variations Subgroup of my Health of the Nation Working Group, chaired by Dr Jeremy Metters, Deputy Chief Medical Officer, has been set up to to prepare a report on how best use can be made of existing information in tackling ethnic, geographical, socio-economic and gender variations in health status (with particular reference to the strength of observed relations and evidence about effectiveness of interventions); to report on areas in which new epidemiological and research information is needed; and to support the Public Health Information Strategy with health variations aspects of its work.

Publication of a consultative document on the organisation of cancer services in England and Wales, and many other initiatives, including projects on ethnic health issues, should help to reduce variations in health and in health care delivery across the country.

To maintain and improve the public health requires constant vigilance, and an intelligence system and organisation which can meet new challenges. To assist with this process the Public Health Network is now well established and a health intelligence officer has been appointed. The Network is connected by computer link (EPINET) and will ensure rapid transfer of information about outbreaks of communicable or non-communicable diseases and other major public health issues. The Inter-Departmental Group on Public Health also provides a forum for discussion of health issues that may be relevant to a wide range of Government Departments and agencies, and many topics have already been discussed.

THE STRATEGY FOR HEALTH

It is now two years since the strategy was launched and its impact continues. An increasing range of organisations and groups now support the strategy, and their energy and enthusiasm continues to grow. My challenge to the nation to improve its health has been taken up by Local Authorities, Government Departments, pharmacies, major stores and other retail outlets, and sports centres. While most of the targets are going in the right direction, three continue to cause concern - cigarette smoking in young people; suicide in young men; and obesity. Continued efforts by all concerned will be required if progress is to be made in these areas.

PROGRESS ON ACTION POINTS IN PREVIOUS REPORTS

A key aspect of these Reports is audit of progress made on issues raised in previous Reports, although for many of the topics identified (including those emphasised this year), action and progress will also depend on individuals and on organisations outside Government Departments and the NHS.

Health of black and ethnic minority groups

An Ethnic Health Unit has now been set up in Leeds by the NHS Executive, and Dr Michael Chan appointed as its Director.

Clinical audit and outcomes of health care

A wide range of initiatives are under way. Health outcomes and knowledge-based care are now seen to be central to effective delivery of health services, and multiprofessional clinical audit is an integral part of care and professional development.

Medical education and manpower

In the first few months of 1994, an initiative was launched on continuing medical education, with strong support from the medical Royal Colleges and deans of postgraduate medical education. A consultation paper has been issued and responses are awaited. This initiative complements progress in undergraduate medical education and in specialist training.

The health of men

A wide variety of local initiatives followed the publication of this special chapter in last year's Report[4]. Conferences, meetings and publications have emphasised the need to consider the particular health problems of men.

Mentally disordered offenders

1993 saw continued emphasis of the need to ensure that services for mentally disordered offenders are taken into account by purchasers and providers of health and social care. Encouraging progress has been made, with a 22.5% increase in the number of patients transferred from prison to inpatient care. Services for mentally disordered offenders were made a high priority in priorities and planning guidance for the NHS in 1994/95[5], and a new committee has met to advise Ministers in the Department of Health (DH) and the Home Office on how to take forward the recommendations of an Inter-Departmental review[6].

Further central capital funding was made available to continue the Medium Secure Unit building programme, which will double the number of places available across the country by mid-1996, and pump-priming money was made available to establish local multi-agency schemes. The National Association for the Care and Resettlement of Offenders (NACRO) was commissioned to prepare a social services training package[7], which will be followed up by six regional seminars.

Verocytotoxin-producing *Escherichia coli*

Verocytotoxin-producing *Escherichia coli* (VTEC) infections associated with food continue to be reported. In May 1993, an outbreak of VTEC 0157, the serogroup which causes most infection, was linked to consumption of raw milk and the micro-organism was isolated from the milk of the implicated herd. This was the first time that VTEC had been isolated from a foodstuff in the United Kingdom (UK). Later in the year, in connection with an outbreak of VTEC infection in Wales, the micro-organism was isolated from a raw beefburger. The Advisory Committee on the Microbiological Safety of Food established a Working Group at the end of 1992 to assess the importance of VTEC as a foodborne pathogen and to advise on any action which could be taken to reduce foodborne diseases associated with it; this Group is expected to report to the Advisory Committee later this year.

NEW ISSUES IDENTIFIED DURING 1993

Each year a small number of issues will be identified as topics of particular importance, to be followed up in subsequent Reports, although the actions needed to ensure progress on these topics may be the responsibility of a wide range of organisations and individuals.

The health of adolescents

Adolescence is the period between childhood and adulthood, and is a crucial period during which lifestyles, values and attitudes are established. Existing health services may not fully cater for their special needs. In general, mortality in this age-group is low: injury and poisoning account for half of all deaths, and three-quarters of all injuries are related to road accidents. Lifestyle issues in this age-group that may set patterns for future life and have long-term effects on health include physical activity, diet, cigarette smoking, alcohol consumption, substance misuse and sexual behaviour. Continuing care for those with chronic diseases (such as cancer, arthritis, diabetes mellitus, asthma or cystic fibrosis), for which treatment begins in childhood but needs to continue in later life, is also of particular concern.

Genetic factors and disease

Genetic factors are of crucial importance in determining health. It has now become possible to identify some genes that are related to particular illnesses and thus to predict, with increasing accuracy, their health implications. The pace of progress continues to accelerate, and it is now possible in some instances to modify a gene or the way in which it expresses its function. Genetic aspects of disease will become increasingly relevant in many areas of health, from screening to treatment, but it is essential to ensure that ethical issues are addressed and that the public, politicians and professionals alike are aware of the implications of these exciting advances. The public health implications of molecular genetics are now with us.

5

Changing patterns of infectious diseases

Despite improvements in immunisation, antibiotics and hygiene, communicable diseases still occur and spread. Not only novel infections, such as HIV/AIDS and VTEC, but older diseases such as tuberculosis, malaria, influenza, and drug-resistant bacteria continue to challenge individual and public health. Outbreaks of infection are still common and inevitable. To combat their effects and to minimise the spread of disease it is essential to have in place a system of surveillance for infectious diseases which identifies any changes at the earliest possible stage. We are fortunate in this country to have the Public Health Laboratory Service which - with its network of laboratories linked to District Directors of Public Health (DDsPH), Consultants in Communicable Disease Control (CsCDC), and Environmental Health Officers (EHOs), and collaborating with 'spotter' general practices and other health care professionals such as health visitors and infection control nurses - provides a comprehensive interlinked system that also takes account of international patterns of infectious diseases. But the public and professionals alike must also ensure that health messages about proper hygiene, correct and appropriate use of antibiotics and immunisation, and avoiding infection (including when travelling abroad) are heeded. Continued vigilance is essential. On 28 July 1994, the Chief Nursing Officer and I announced plans[8] to offer protection against measles and rubella to all 5-15-year-old children through an intensive immunisation programme in November 1994; this initiative is designed to prevent a predicted epidemic of measles in the next few years, and to allow the school rubella vaccination programme to be stopped.

Asthma

The past decade has seen a striking increase in hospital admissions and general practitioner (GP) consultations for asthma, which affects over 2 million people including some 500,000 below the age of 16 years, and causes over 1,600 deaths annually. Asthma is the result of an allergic response to foreign material which affects the lungs and causes wheezing and difficulty in breathing; there may often be a genetic predisposition to the illness, which can be triggered by various factors including diet, maternal cigarette smoking, and indoor and outdoor air pollution. Research continues into the causes of and most effective treatments for asthma, and recent initiatives include the introduction of chronic disease management programmes in general practice, the use of treatment guidelines and a role for specialist nurses. There has also been particular emphasis on possible effects of air pollution. Indoor allergens (such as the house dust mite) appear to have increased over the past 20 years, possibly related to central heating, fitted carpets and improved insulation. The effects of outdoor air pollution are being extensively studied and over the next year several reports into issues related to air pollution and asthma should help to identify scientific evidence for a possible link between air pollution and asthma, and put any such link into context.

EXECUTIVE SUMMARY

VITAL STATISTICS

Population size

The resident population of England at 30 June 1993 was 48.5 million, an increase of 0.3% compared with 1992.

Age and sex structure of the resident population

The pre-school and school-age populations are fairly stable. The younger working population aged 16-29 years is falling whereas the older working population (aged 30-59 years for women and 30-64 years for men) is increasing. There is still a rapid increase in the number of people aged 85 years and over, three-quarters of whom are women.

Fertility statistics - aspects of relevance for health care

In 1991, 808,989 conceptions occurred to women resident in England. The overall conception rate reached 77.8 per 1,000 women aged 15-44 years in 1991. The conception rate among females aged under 16 years was 9.3 per 1,000 aged 13-15 years, a fall of 7% compared with 1990. There were an estimated 640,000 live births in England in 1993, 2% less than in 1992.

Mortality

There were estimated to be 544,000 deaths registered in England in 1993, 4% more than in 1992. The crude mortality rate increased from 10.8 per 1,000 in 1992 to 11.1 in 1993.

There was an outbreak of influenza in the autumn of 1993, which was thought to be responsible for a greater than expected number of deaths from October to the end of the year.

Prevalence of disease in the community

In 1991/92, 78% of all National Health Service (NHS) patients consulted in general practice. The highest proportions of consultations were among children aged less than 5 years, and people aged over 65 years. Respiratory diseases accounted for more consultations than any other group of diseases.

In 1992, 32% of respondents to the General Household Survey (GHS) reported a long-standing illness, 19% a limiting long-standing illness and 12% restricted activity in the two weeks before the interview. The prevalence of reported long-standing illness increased during the 1980s, but has remained fairly constant since the end of that decade.

7

Infant and perinatal mortality

In 1992 in England, 4,259 babies died before the age of one year. The infant mortality rate was 6.5 per 1,000 live births, the lowest ever recorded. 2,975 stillbirths were recorded in 1992.

Trends in cancer incidence

For all malignant neoplasms combined (excluding non-melanoma skin cancer), there was an increase in incidence over the period 1979-89. Lung cancer registration decreased among males but increased for females over this period. Overall cancer mortality has shown no decline in recent years, but there has been a fall in the mortality rate for cancer of the stomach for both sexes.

Trends in reporting congenital malformations

According to provisional data for 1993, the number of malformed live births decreased by 6% between 1992 and 1993, from 5,618 to 5,292.

THE NATION'S HEALTH

Public health in England

The national Public Health Network continued to draw together public health skills and specialist knowledge to advance the public health. Surveillance of the public health function continued, and a working party chaired by Dr Michael Abrams, formerly Deputy Chief Medical Officer, reported on the public health responsibilities of the NHS and others in November[9]. Communicable disease control, funding for public health training and the role of nursing professionals in public health are under review.

Inter-Departmental Group on Public Health

The Inter-Departmental Group on Public Health reviews health issues across a wide range of Government Departments.

Sickness at work

Avoidable ill-health is a burden not only to the NHS but also to employers. The need for effective health care and counselling for employees needs to be emphasised, as well as the requirement to ensure safety.

Urban health

Urbanisation may have many effects, including overcrowding, poor housing and sanitation, and pollution. Many of these are relevant to health and the provision of health services.

Variations in health

Variations in health may be observed in relation to geographical area, ethnicity, social class, occupation and gender. The steps that the NHS might take to reduce these variations are being reviewed in relation to key area targets in the strategy for health.

Health of people in later life

In the 'European Year of Older People and Solidarity between Generations', progress was made towards more effective delivery of care to elderly people.

Health of black and ethnic minorities

An Ethnic Health Unit was established by the NHS Management Executive. Further surveys and research into issues related to the health needs of black and ethnic minorities were continued.

Health of men

Although many of the major causes of death and illness are similar in men and women alike, men have specific health and health care needs which should be recognised.

THE STRATEGY FOR HEALTH

One year on

Following publication of *The Health of the Nation*[1] in July 1992, a review of progress was summarised in the report *One Year On*[10], published in November 1993. In July 1993, the Chief Medical Officer issued a challenge to the nation to take some of 20 simple steps that could be taken by individuals to improve their own health.

Key areas and targets

Coronary heart disease and stroke: Risk factors for coronary heart disease (CHD) and stroke were analysed in the report of the 1991 Health Survey for England[11], published in July 1993, and will be monitored in subsequent years.

Cancers: Progress continues towards meeting published targets for breast, cervical, skin and lung cancer, although cigarette smoking among children aged 11-15 years is still too high.

Mental illness: Assessment of how to measure the main targets continues to be refined, and policy on the care of people with severe and enduring mental illness was comprehensively reviewed, with the announcement of a ten-point plan to reinforce community care for mentally ill people.

HIV/AIDS and sexual health: Work continues to sustain progress towards targets in this key area, with initiatives for HIV prevention and sexual health promotion, and to combat drug misuse. NHS health authorities are required to provide a full range of family planning services.

Accidents: Encouraging progress has been made towards mortality targets, but injuries caused by accidents far exceed deaths. The range and compatibility of information collected about accidental injuries is one of the main priorities of the national Accident Prevention Task Force.

Nutrition

The Nutrition Task Force issued an outline programme of action for public consultation; a final programme was adopted in the light of comments received and will be published in Spring 1994. A National Breast-feeding Working Group first met in 1993. A Nutrition Programme Committee oversaw a call for research proposals in nutrition, and successful proposals were commissioned in December.

Implementation

NHS activities: The improvement of public health through implementation of the Health of the Nation strategy was identified as one of the top priorities for the NHS in its *Priorities and Planning Guidance 1994/95*[5]. Regional Health Authorities (RHAs) have produced plans to implement the strategy, with local health goals to take account of local needs and variations in health. The Health at Work in the NHS initiative continues to promote the health of staff in the NHS.

Local health alliances: Local health alliances to set local strategies for health continue to be encouraged.

Healthy settings: The concept of 'healthy settings' - cities, schools, hospitals, the workplace, homes, the environment and prisons - is being supported and developed.

Inter-Departmental co-operation: A Cabinet committee co-ordinates the implementation, monitoring and development of the strategy for health across different Government Departments.

The way ahead

Continued support for health promotion will include an awards scheme and further work with the Department for Education in schools and colleges, and with health professionals in primary care.

HEALTH OF ADOLESCENTS

Adolescence is the transitional phase between childhood and adulthood, characterised by experimentation and rapid change. This is a key time for individuals to establish health-related values, attitudes and lifestyles - which may have longstanding positive or negative influences on future health.

Mortality

Injury and poisoning accounted for over half the total deaths among young adolescents in England and Wales in 1992, followed by neoplasms and diseases of the nervous system. Respiratory diseases were the fourth biggest killer in 1982, but had fallen by 1992 to less than 1 death per 100,000 population.

Morbidity

Routine statistics do not provide specific evidence of adolescent disease profiles, but consultation rates in general practice appear to be broadly similar to those for adults aged 25-64 years although hospital admission rates are lower at 10-14 years and 15-19 years than for most 5-year age-groups.

Specific conditions

Injury: Road traffic accidents account for three-quarters of accidental deaths in 15-24-year-olds.

Cancer: Hodgkin's disease and lymphomas (22%), leukaemias (16%) and brain tumours (14%) account for more than half of the 900 new cases of cancer reported annually in people aged 10-19 years.

Diabetes mellitus: The prevalence of diabetes mellitus in adolescents is about 2 per 1,000 population, and accounts for about 0.6% of hospital admissions.

Asthma: General practitioner (GP) consultations for asthma have increased over the past 10 years, although this finding may reflect improved diagnosis. Symptoms and care requirements in adolescents are similar to those in the whole population, but the psychological effects of chronic illness in adolescence may be greater than in older age-groups.

Sexually transmitted diseases: About one-third of reports of post-pubertal uncomplicated gonorrhoea in females are in those aged 19 years and under.

Dental health: Dental health in adolescents continues to improve; in 1993, only 48% of 15-year-olds had fillings, compared with 85% in 1983.

Lifestyle and health

Health and lifestyle factors play a major role in many conditions that cause morbidity and mortality in later life. Establishment of a healthy lifestyle during adolescence has wide-ranging benefits.

Physical activity: There has been concern about low levels of physical activity in young people, but in one local survey over 80% of 14-year-olds claimed to take some form of regular exercise.

Diet and nutrition: Diet and nutrient intakes of British schoolchildren in 1983 were similar to those in adults, although there was some evidence of low calcium and iron intakes in adolescent girls.

Smoking: Adult smoking prevalence continues to fall but 1992 figures for cigarette smoking in 11-15-year-olds are virtually unchanged at 10%. Health education campaigns have been broadened to involve parents in tackling this problem.

Alcohol misuse: Regular drinking often begins at an early age and weekly consumption in 14-15-year-olds appears to be increasing. The recommended sensible drinking limits for adults may not be applicable to adolescents, and the proportion drinking in excess of them gives cause for concern.

Substance misuse: Most young people never try to misuse drugs, but the numbers who do, and the wide availability of drugs open to misuse, give no grounds for complacency.

Sexual behaviour: The number of adolescent pregnancies is still a cause for concern, although conception rates fell in 1991. Effective sex education and the availability of confidential counselling and contraception are essential to reduce the traumas caused by adolescent pregnancy or termination of pregnancy.

Mental health: Depression and suicidal thoughts are common in adolescence; more females than males attempt self harm, but suicide is commoner in young males - among whom suicide rates have risen recently against overall national trends.

Social factors

Child protection: The incidence of child abuse is not known precisely, but increased public awareness and professional recognition have led to increased reporting and identification.

Children looked after by Local Authorities: Most children looked after by Local Authorities are in foster homes, reflecting a move away from care in children's homes.

Divorce: The divorce rate in England is among the highest in Europe, and on present trends one in four children will experience breakdown in their parents' marriage by the age of 16 years.

Violence: Most of our knowledge of patterns of violent behaviour in adolescents comes from the United States of America, but the problem appears to be related to environment, family breakdown, poverty, social control (or lack of it), and individual psychological make-up.

Unauthorised school absence: In 1992-93, 12% of young people in maintained secondary schools had engaged in unauthorised absence at least once. Such absences may lead to health and behavioural, as well as educational, difficulties.

Employment: Adolescent unemployment has been higher than the general level of unemployment over the past 20 years. The effects of part-time jobs whilst still at school, or of parental unemployment, are not fully established.

Homelessness: Adolescents may be homeless in their own right, or as part of a homeless family. In the 1991 Census, 2,439 people under 18 years-of-age in England were sleeping rough or in lodging houses or hostels.

Health services for adolescents

Adolescents may have particular needs for health services distinct from those of children or adults, and there is also a need to ensure continuity of care for those adolescents with chronic illness who will need to transfer from paediatric to adult hospital services.

Improving the health of adolescents

Many determinants of adolescent health are behavioural and lifestyle-related, and may be amenable to intervention. Encouragingly, most adolescents seem to recognise that some aspects of health are largely self-determined and a matter of personal responsibility.

HEALTH CARE

Needs, effectiveness and outcomes

Assessing health care needs: Health needs assessment is the main activity upon which cost-effective purchasing is based. To support this, epidemiologically based needs reviews continue to be published, and a project to look at the assessment of health needs at local level has been set up.

Basic sources of information: DH's programme of surveys continued to evolve during 1993, with surveys of cardiovascular disease, psychiatric morbidity and diet and nutrition in toddlers. Substantial progress has also been made in developing the NHS Management Executive's information management and technology strategy[12].

National confidential enquiries: The five national confidential enquiries continued to make good progress. It is important that the recommendations of such enquiries are implemented to improve the quality and outcome of care in their respective fields.

Quality of service and effectiveness of care: 1993 has been a year of transition, with completion of a move from uniprofessional to multiprofessional audit and emphasis of the need to establish clinical audit as an integral part of normal clinical practice.

Clinical standards and guidelines: DHAs and GP fundholders continue to develop more sophisticated approaches to purchasing health care on the basis of information about the effectiveness of clinical interventions.

Clinical audit in primary care: Clinical multidisciplinary audit should be an integral part of continuing professional development, and its educational value is becoming increasingly recognised.

Health outcomes: Central initiatives to take forward the concept of health outcomes of care continue to evolve. During 1993, DH published a consultation document on the first set of population health outcome indicators for the NHS[13]. After consultation, work has now started on the development of further indicators.

Primary health care

Organisation of primary care: Primary and community care has a major role as patient health services evolve through NHS reforms. 1993 saw the implementation of *Caring for People*[14], a widening of GP fundholder purchasing, further improvements in cervical cytology and childhood vaccination coverage, and a focusing of health promotion in general practice[15].

Prescribing: The real costs of prescribing continue to rise but educational initiatives should help doctors to deliver high-quality but cost-effective health care.

Professional development: Continuing professional development is vital for the delivery of high-quality primary health care, encouraged by continuing education and training programmes, clinical audit and assistance to practices.

The way ahead: Challenges ahead for GPs and other members of primary care teams will include the need to deliver an increasing range of services in a community setting whilst still meeting existing demands for primary health services.

Hospital services

Specialised services: The needs of patients who require certain specialised services were investigated by the Clinical Standards Advisory Group (CSAG)[16,17]. Streamlined arrangements for purchasing of tertiary extra-contractual referrals were introduced in February[18], and advice on contracting for specialised services was issued in November[19].

Cancer: An Expert Advisory Group on cancer was established by the Chief Medical Officers of England and Wales.

National Confidential Enquiry into Peri-operative Deaths: The National Confidential Enquiry into Peri-operative Deaths (NCEPOD) issued its report for 1991/92 during 1993[20].

Diabetes mellitus

The first report from the joint DH/British Diabetic Association (BDA) St Vincent Task Force for Diabetes was accepted by DH Ministers and the BDA Executive Council in July.

Asthma

Asthma sufficiently severe to require regular medical supervision affects 4-6% of children and about 4% of adults. Admissions to hospital and prescription costs have increased. The causes of increased prevalence are not understood, but maternal smoking and allergy, particularly to house dust mite, are relevant.

Osteopathy and chiropractic

The Osteopathy Act 1993, which provides a legislative framework for the regulation of osteopathy by a General Osteopathic Council, received Royal Assent in July[21]. A Private Member's Bill to establish a similar legislative framework for the regulation of chiropractic has been introduced by Mr David Lidington MP.

Mental health

Mental health and primary care: Primary care provides considerable opportunities to achieve the mental health targets of the Health of the Nation initiative[1], and DH continues to support several projects.

Occupational mental health: The importance of mental health in occupational settings continued to be emphasised, supported by a conference on promoting mental health policies in the workplace, publication of a booklet for employers[22] and inclusion of mental health of the NHS workforce as one of six NHS research and development priorities in mental health.

Services for people with severe mental illness: In August, the Secretary of State for Health announced the findings of a review of legal powers on the care of mentally ill people in the community[23], which concluded that a power of supervised discharge should supplement existing powers[24]. A ten-point plan for developing safe and successful community care was also announced[25].

Services for mentally disordered offenders: Following publication of the review of services for mentally disordered offenders[6], a second national needs assessment exercise was completed. Services, particularly schemes diverting patients from the criminal justice system to health and social care, have been greatly expanded, with a substantial increase in patients transferring from prison to health care.

Mental health legislation: A team set up to review whether new legal powers were needed to ensure that mentally ill people in the community get the care they need reported in August, with recommendations for some amendments to the Mental Health Act 1983[24].

Maternity and child health services

Report of the Expert Maternity Group: The Expert Maternity Group's report[26] *Changing Childbirth*, was published for consultation in August.

Confidential Enquiries into Maternal Deaths: The Report on Confidential Enquiries into Maternal Deaths in the United Kingdom (UK), 1988-1990, was prepared and will be published early in 1994.

Folic acid and neural tube defects: The Report of an Expert Advisory Group and guidance from the UK Health Departments' Chief Medical Officers were widely distributed, and a public education poster and leaflet were prepared.

Vitamin A and pregnancy: The Chief Medical Officer confirmed earlier advice that women who are pregnant or who might become pregnant should not consume liver or excessive amounts of vitamin A supplements[27].

Human Fertilisation and Embryology Authority: The Human Fertilisation and Embryology Authority (HFEA) continues to address contentious ethical issues by seeking public responses to consultation documents[28,29].

Sudden infant death syndrome: The extended report of the Expert Group on Sleeping Position of Infants and Cot Death was published[30], and a summary of the evidence and of the Group's recommendations and conclusions were sent to health professionals by the Chief Medical and Nursing Officers[31].

Prophylaxis of vitamin K deficiency bleeding in infants: DH commissioned further studies into the reported association between use of intramuscular vitamin K in infants and childhood cancer, as noted in last year's Report[32]. Further studies in Sweden[33] and the USA[34] were unable to verify any such association.

Neonatal intensive care: The CSAG report *Access to and Availability of Specialised Services*[16] included the report of a group set up to consider neonatal intensive care[35].

Paediatric intensive care: The British Paediatric Association's multidisciplinary report on paediatric intensive care was published in November[36].

Confidential Enquiry into Stillbirths and Deaths in Infancy: The Confidential Enquiry into Stillbirths and Deaths in Infancy (CESDI) completed its first programme of enquiries during 1993 and the National Advisory Body that guides CESDI submitted its first Annual Report to Ministers, including early results from its rapid reporting system, in November[37].

Notification of congenital malformations: The Office of Population Censuses and Surveys (OPCS) notification system to monitor congenital malformations, introduced in 1964, is being reviewed.

Gene Therapy Advisory Committee: During 1993, the Secretary of State for Health established a new non-statutory body, the Gene Therapy Advisory Committee (GTAC). GTAC succeeds the Committee on the Ethics of Gene Therapy (the Clothier Committee).

Learning disabilities

After publication of the report *Services for People with Learning Disabilities and Challenging Behaviour or Mental Health Needs*[38], an Advisory Group and a National Implementation Network were set up to encourage and oversee progress in fulfilling the needs of people with learning disabilities who have behavioural disturbance or mental health needs.

Disability and rehabilitation

During 1993, developments in the fields of disability, rehabilitation and audiology included the Public Accounts Committee's[39] consideration of the National Audit Office Report on Health Services for Physically Disabled People aged 16 to 64 years[40], inclusion of the need to ensure appropriate local services for disabled people as one of the priorities for the NHS for 1994/95[5], and an initiative on pressure sores, as well as other developments in research and medical education about various aspects of disability or rehabilitation.

Prison health care

The Prison Service became an Executive Agency of the Home Office in April and launched several initiatives to ensure that prisoners receive the same range and quality of health care services as the general public.

COMMUNICABLE DISEASES

HIV infection and AIDS

Data reported for HIV infection and AIDS showed a similar pattern to previous years. In 1993, they were combined with data from unlinked anonymous surveillance as a basis for a new report on projections for infection in England and Wales up to 1997[41]. Publication of the new report was accompanied by a statement of Government strategy on HIV/AIDS, which reaffirms commitment to this area.

In 1993, DH issued guidance on notifying patients of HIV-infected health care workers[42], and interim guidelines on the management of HIV-infected health care workers[43].

Other sexually transmitted diseases

The total number of new cases seen at genito-urinary medicine clinics continues to rise, although the proportion actually diagnosed as having a sexually transmitted disease (STD) fell in 1992 and the number of reports of many STDs decreased. A fall in the total reports of gonorrhoea by just under 24% resulted in an incidence below the target set by the Health of the Nation initiative[1]. Exceptions to the general downward trend were pelvic inflammatory disease and first attacks of herpes simplex; reports of recurrent herpes simplex and recurrent viral warts also increased. A significant proportion of the reports of STDs were from younger age-groups, particularly among women.

Immunisation

Immunisation coverage continues to rise and increasing numbers of DHAs are now reaching 95% coverage for all childhood immunisations. The impact of the introduction of vaccine against *Haemophilus influenzae* type b (Hib) infection has been impressive: laboratory reports of meningitis and septicaemia caused by this micro-organism at all ages have fallen by almost two-thirds, and the reduction in children under one year-of-age is close to 85%.

Hepatitis B guidelines

New guidelines for protecting health care workers and patients from hepatitis B were issued by the NHS Management Executive[44].

Influenza

Influenza activity occurred early in the Autumn of 1993 before the annual immunisation of at-risk patients had been completed.

Tuberculosis

In April 1993, the World Health Organization (WHO) declared tuberculosis to be a global emergency. Notifications continued to rise in many European countries, including the UK. DH established an Inter-Departmental Task Force to consider and to take forward necessary action and guidance.

Foodborne and waterborne diseases

Notifications of food poisoning continued to increase, but to a lesser degree than in 1992. By contrast, the number of reports of salmonellosis, campylobacter enteritis and listeriosis remained at much the same level as for the previous year, and the number of isolations of verocytotoxin-producing *Escherichia coli*

(VTEC) 0157 decreased. The Advisory Committee on the Microbiological Safety of Food is assessing the significance of VTEC as a foodborne pathogen and will advise on any action to be taken to reduce associated disease. During 1993, VTEC 0157, the principal serogroup causing human illness, was isolated from food in the UK for the first time.

Travel-related disease

In view of increasing reports of diphtheria from the Russian Federation and the Ukraine, the Chief Medical Officer recommended that travellers to these areas should be immunised against diphtheria[45]. New guidelines for prophylaxis against malaria for travellers from the UK were published[46].

ENVIRONMENTAL HEALTH AND TOXICOLOGY

Chemical and physical agents in the environment

Small Area Health Statistics Unit: The Small Area Health Statistics Unit made good progress during 1993. Several major studies of health statistics in the vicinity of point sources of industrial pollution, including a petrochemical works and municipal incinerators, are nearing completion and will be published shortly. Advances in the methodology for investigating health statistics in small areas have been made.

Air pollution episodes: The Department of the Environment's Expert Panel on Air Quality Standards, which has a joint secretariat with DH, will publish recommendations for an air quality standard for benzene in Spring 1994. Work on a standard for ozone and 1,3-butadiene was begun in 1993 and work on sulphur dioxide is well advanced; recommendations will be made in 1994, and standards for oxides of nitrogen, particles and polycyclic aromatic hydrocarbon compounds will follow.

Institute for Environment and Health: The Institute for Environment and Health was established by the Medical Research Council with the support of the Departments of Health and the Environment.

NHS response to chemical accidents: Guidance was issued to Health Authorities on the health aspects of chemical contamination incidents[47].

Distribution of stable iodine: New guidance regarding stable iodine tablets for use in the event of a nuclear emergency was published[48,49].

Toxicological safety

Food hazards and food hygiene education: The emergency system deals quickly and effectively with chemical emergencies and can be contacted for toxicological advice on a 24-hour basis.

Food carcinogen prioritisation: Work continued on the prioritisation of chemical contaminants in food based on the carcinogenic risk they pose to the population. Different methods of allowing for carcinogenic potency have been considered.

Mineral hydrocarbons in food: Further action on mineral hydrocarbons are being considered and need to be integrated into European Community (EC) actions.

Advisory Committee on Novel Foods and Processes: The Committee's role in allowing only safe novel foods onto the market continues to increase.

Pesticide residues in food: People in certain areas were advised to restrict their consumption of eels, because of organochlorine pesticide residues[50].

Veterinary drugs: Ministers decided that Departments responsible for animal feedingstuffs should regularly review new developments.

Sheep dips and occupational health: Reports of adverse reactions to organophosphorus compounds used to dip sheep led the Veterinary Products Committee to review these preparations in 1993, with the result that a system of certification will be introduced for sheep dippers.

MEDICAL EDUCATION, TRAINING AND STAFFING

Junior doctors' hours

1993 saw the elimination of nearly all posts where junior doctors were contracted for over 83 hours a week, creating a strong framework within which to make further progress.

'Achieving a Balance'

Medical staffing policy focused on the reduction of junior doctors' hours and consequent modifications to this initiative.

Medical Manpower Standing Advisory Committee

Recommendations of the first report of the Medical Manpower Standing Advisory Committee, published in December 1992[51], were accepted. A second report is expected towards the end of 1994.

Equal opportunities for doctors

Several new initiatives were announced on equality issues, particularly on improving access to, and opportunities for, flexible training and on setting new goals for doctors from ethnic minorities.

Part-time consultant scheme

Eighty five new, centrally funded posts were approved under a scheme to promote part-time opportunities at consultant level[52].

New career structure for doctors in community health

Negotiations on the establishment of a combined child health service were completed, and guidance will be issued early in 1994.

Postgraduate, continuing and specialist medical and dental education

In December, Ministers announced[53] that the recommendations of the Working Party Report on Specialist Medical Training[54] had been accepted. Interim arrangements were introduced in April for the funding of hospital medical and dental training posts, and GP clinical tutors became eligible for sessional payments as part of the postgraduate deans' regional education network.

Undergraduate medical and dental education

The Steering Group on Undergraduate Medical and Dental Education and Research published its third report[55]. Funding was provided to medical schools to facilitate the introduction of General Medical Council (GMC) recommendations for change in undergraduate medical education.

Doctors' performance

The Review's early discussions identified certain issues - such as unacceptable behaviour, poor communication, attitudinal aspects and education - as issues for further consideration and a report is expected in 1994.

Locum doctors

A Working Group to examine ways to ensure quality control of locum doctors working in the NHS is due to report in Autumn 1994.

OTHER TOPICS OF INTEREST IN 1993

Medicines Control Agency

Role and performance: The role of the Medicines Control Agency (MCA) is to protect the public health by ensuring that all medicines for human use meet satisfactory standards of safety, quality and efficacy. The MCA met most of its targets, reduced licensing times, eliminated backlogs and achieved Trading Fund status during the year.

Control of UK clinical trials: The MCA proposes to introduce new procedures to ease the administrative burden associated with authorisation of clinical trials, without compromising the safety of patient volunteers.

Reclassification of medicines from Prescription Only to Pharmacy status: The MCA has speeded up the procedure for reclassifying Prescription Only Medicines to allow over-the-counter supply from pharmacies, although safety remains the criterion to determine whether a medicine can move from prescription control. A record number of requests for changes were handled during the year.

Control of gene therapy products: Gene therapy is an emerging area of medicine with the potential to provide effective treatments for genetic diseases, cancer and immune diseases. Existing UK and EC legislation covers nearly all the aspects of gene therapy products but close co-operation with other Government advisory bodies and departments will be necessary to ensure their safe clinical use.

Developments in the European Community: The MCA continues to implement a number of EC Directives. Its main work during the year centred upon the preparations for the introduction of a new European drug regulatory system.

European Medicines Evaluation Agency

The EC adopted legislation setting out the new EC licensing arrangements (Future Systems) and agreed that the new European Medicines Evaluation Agency should be sited in London. It will co-ordinate the activities of national licensing authorities.

National Blood Authority

The National Blood Authority was set up on 1 April, taking over the roles of the Central Blood Laboratories Authority and the National Directorate of the National Blood Transfusion Service.

Creutzfeldt-Jakob disease surveillance

A surveillance unit for Creutzfeldt-Jakob disease (CJD) was set up in Edinburgh in 1990; the annual incidence of CJD in the UK reflects the worldwide distribution of 0.5-1 per million population. A report from Australia[56] indicated a possible link between the occurrence of CJD and parenteral treatment with human pituitary gonadotrophin derived from cadavers. An advice centre to trace and offer counselling for the few women who received similar treatment in the UK between 1956 and 1985 was set up[57].

Medical devices

The Medical Devices Directorate (MDD) continued to monitor the safety and efficacy of medical devices and to implement EC Directives for statutory regulation of medical devices. During 1993, MDD received over 2,700 reports of problems, investigated half of these reports in depth, and issued 12 Hazard Notices and 40 Safety Action Bulletins.

Bioethics

Local Research Ethics Committees: During the year, DH consulted widely on appropriate training for members of Local Research Ethics Committees (LRECs) and ways to streamline procedures for multicentre research.

Bioethics in Europe: The Council of Europe's Steering Committee on Bioethics (CDBI) continued to develop proposals for a framework bioethics convention.

Committee on the Ethics of Gene Therapy: After wide consultation, Ministers accepted the recommendations of the Clothier Committee and announced the establishment of the Gene Therapy Advisory Committee.

Ethics of genetic screening: The Nuffield Council on Bioethics Working Party's report on ethical issues associated with genetic screening was published[58]. The reaction of public and professional interests is being assessed.

Lifestyle and treatment: Inappropriate or insensitive expression by doctors of personal views on spiritual or moral, rather than medical grounds, is being reviewed by the GMC.

London Implementation Group

February saw the publication of *Making London Better*[59] the Government's response to Professor Sir Bernard Tomlinson's inquiry into London's health services, medical education and research[60]. The London Implementation Group was formed to take forward, in conjunction with existing health agencies, the strategy for change it contained.

Research and development

Report of the Advisory Council on Science and Technology: The Government welcomed[61] the report on medical research and health of the Advisory Council on Science and Technology[62].

White Paper on Science and Technology: This major policy review of science and technology was launched in May[63], and has led to several initiatives.

Research for health: The report *Research for Health*[64], published in June, summarised progress and set the direction of DH's research and development strategy.

Dental health

Dental health of the nation: The dental health of the nation continues to improve, although the rate of improvement among children may have levelled off. Children in some inner-city areas and members of some ethnic minority groups may be at increased risk of dental caries.

General dental services: Sir Kenneth Bloomfield's report[65] into remuneration of general dental practitioners, and options for change, was followed by wide consultation. In June, the House of Commons Health Select Committee published its report into dental services[66].

Community dental services: Statistics collection Form KC64 for community dental services was revised during 1993. The new form will be introduced after further planning and consultation.

Hospital dental services: The number of hospital dentists in England rose by 4.6% between September 1991 and September 1992. New outpatient referrals to consultant clinics rose in 1992/93 compared with 1991/92.

Continuing education and training for dentists: Vocational training schemes for general dental services (GDS) continued to expand. By 1 October, all dentists applying for inclusion in Family Health Services Authority lists of practitioners who have agreed to provide GDS must have taken part in such a scheme or obtained exemption.

Dental research: Dental research commissioned by DH included a study of the dental needs of elderly people, research into the dental health of children registered in the NHS capitation scheme and a study to evaluate a radiographic quality assurance programme.

INTERNATIONAL HEALTH

Britain, Europe and health

The UK faces many of the same health challenges as its near neighbours in Europe, and continues to work with them, particularly in the EC, the Council of Europe, and the WHO. In the EC, progress is being made towards a more coherent and consistent approach to public health, with the publication of the Commission's Framework for Action in the Field of Public Health. This lays down a basis on which Member States can debate co-operation over key challenges such as cancer and communicable diseases.

The European Community

Treaty of European Union (Maastricht): The Maastricht Treaty, with its provisions on public health, is now firmly in force.

European Economic Area: The European institutional background continues to develop, with the establishment of the European Economic Area and negotiations for the accession of four new Member States.

EC/WHO/Council of Europe Co-operation: Close co-operation between EC, WHO and the Council of Europe continued during 1993.

Free movement of people: EC Regulations to co-ordinate the health care schemes of Member States continue to operate effectively.

Directive on data protection: Discussions continued in an Internal Market Council Working Party on a draft EC Directive on Data Protection.

Smoking: The Health Council considered a number of possible measures to help reduce smoking.

Elderly and disabled people: 1993 was the 'European Year of Older People and Solidarity between Generations' and saw the adoption of HELIOS II, the third Community action programme for disabled people.

AIDS and HIV infection: The UK continued to be active in work on HIV and AIDS and supported a number of initiatives on World International AIDS Day.

Pharmaceuticals: A new Pharmaceutical Price Regulation Scheme was agreed, and this met the requirements of Directive 89/105/EEC.

Research and information technology: DH continues to be involved in the EC's research programmes.

Food safety: The General Food Hygiene Directive was adopted in June 1993, and was an important achievement of the UK Presidency of the EC.

Relations with Central and Eastern Europe

The UK continued to foster links with Central and Eastern Europe and to offer assistance to health programmes in times of change for these countries. DH has Health Co-operation Agreements with a number of countries in Central and Eastern Europe. DH and the NHS also responded to requests from the United Nations High Commission for Refugees for treatment to be given to medical evacuees from Bosnia and Croatia.

Council of Europe

The UK was active in the Council of Europe's European Health Committee and its Bioethics Committee, and UK experts participated in select committees and working groups covering a range of current health issues.

The Commonwealth

The Chief Medical Officer led a delegation to the Commonwealth Health Ministers' meeting which preceded the World Health Assembly.

World Health Organization

European Regional Committee: In September, the European Regional Committee appointed a Standing Committee to facilitate interaction between itself and the Copenhagen Secretariat. Regional priorities were set up to 2001 and a Search Committee was established to identify suitable candidates to contest the 1995 Regional Director election.

Executive Board: In January, the WHO Executive Board recommended the re-election of Dr Hiroshi Nakajima as Director-General, a decision endorsed by the World Health Assembly which re-elected Dr Nakajima in May.

World Health Assembly: The Board and the Assembly strongly supported the recommendations of the Working Group, chaired by the Chief Medical Officer, on Global Reform in WHO. The main item on the World Health Assembly agenda was the Organization's programme budget for the 1994/95 biennium.

References

1. Department of Health. *The Health of the Nation: a strategy for health in England.* London: HMSO, 1992 (Cm. 1986).
2. Department of Health. *On the State of the Public Health: the annual report of the Chief Medical Officer of the Department of Health for the year 1992.* London: HMSO, 1993; 2.
3. Department of Health. Influenza immunisation. *CMO's Update* 1993; **3**: 1-2.
4. Department of Health. *On the State of the Public Health: the annual report of the Chief Medical Officer of the Department of Health for the year 1992.* London: HMSO, 1993; 6, 79-106.
5. NHS Executive. *Priorities and planning guidance for the NHS in 1994/95.* Heywood (Lancashire): Department of Health 1993 (Executive Letter: EL(93)54).
6. Department of Health, Home Office. *Review of health and social services for mentally disordered offenders and others requiring similar services: final summary report.* London: HMSO, 1992 (Cm. 2088).
7. National Association for the Care and Resettlement of Offenders, Department of Health. *Working with Mentally Disordered Offenders: a training pack for social services staff and others.* London: NACRO, 1994.
8. Department of Health. *National Measles and Rubella Vaccination Campaign.* Heywood (Lancashire): Department of Health, 1994 (Professional Letter: PL/CMO(94)10, PL/CNO(94)13).
9. Department of Health, Department of Environment. *Public Health responsibilities of the NHS and roles of others.* Heywood (Lancashire): Department of Health, 1993 (Miscellaneous Circular: MISC (93)56).
10. Department of Health. *Health of the Nation: one year on - a report on the progress of the Health of the Nation.* London: Department of Health, 1993.
11. Office of Population Censuses and Surveys. *Health Survey for England 1991.* London: HMSO, 1993.
12. Department of Health. *An Information Management and Technology Strategy for the NHS in England: IM&T Strategy Overview.* Cambridge: Information Management Group of the NHS Management Executive, 1992.
13. Department of Health. *Population Health Outcomes Indicators for the NHS: 1993 England: a consultation document.* London: Department of Health, 1993.
14. Department of Health. *Caring for People.* London: Department of Health, 1993.
15. Department of Health. *New worlds, new opportunities: nursing in primary health care.* Heywood (Lancashire): Department of Health, 1993.
16. Clinical Standards Advisory Group. *Access to and Availability of Specialist Services: report of a CSAG committee.* London: HMSO, 1993. Chair: Professor John Richmond.
17. Department of Health. *Government response to the reports by the Clinical Standards Advisory Group on Access to and Availability of Specialist Services.* Heywood (Lancashire): Department of Health, 1993.
18. Department of Health. *Guidance on operation of notification arrangements for tertiary extra-contractual referrals.* Heywood (Lancashire): Department of Health, 1993 (Health Service Guidelines: HSG(93)8).
19. Department of Health. *Contracting for specialised services.* Heywood (Lancashire): Department of Health, 1993 (Executive Letter: EL(93)98).
20. Campling GA, Devlin HB, Hoile RW et al. *The Report of the National Confidential Enquiry into Peri-operative Deaths 1991/92.* London: National Confidential Enquiry into Peri-operative Deaths, 1993.
21. *Osteopathy Act 1993.* London: HMSO, 1993.
22. Department of Health. *Mental Illness: a guide to mental health in the workplace.* London: Department of Health, 1993.
23. Department of Health. *Legal powers on the care of mentally ill people in the community.* London: Department of Health, 1993.
24. *Mental Health Act 1983.* London: HMSO, 1983.
25. Department of Health. *Legislation planned to provide for supervised discharge of psychiatric patients.* London: Department of Health, 1993 (Press Release: H93/908).
26. Department of Health. *Changing Childbirth: part 1: report of the Expert Maternity Group.* London: HMSO, 1993. Chair: Baroness Cumberlege.

27. Department of Health. *Vitamin A and pregnancy.* Heywood (Lancashire): Department of Health, 1993 (Professional Letter: PL/CMO(93)15).

28. *Human Fertilisation and Embryology Authority Code of Practice (Revised 1993).* London: Human Fertilisation and Embryology Authority, 1993.

29. Human Fertilisation and Embryology Authority. *Sex selection: public consultation document.* London: Human Fertilisation and Embryology Authority, 1993.

30. Department of Health. *Report of the Chief Medical Officer's Expert Group on the Sleeping Positions of Infants and Cot Death.* London: HMSO, 1993. Chair: Dr Eileen Rubery.

31. Department of Health. *Cot Death.* Heywood (Lancashire): Department of Health, 1993 (Professional Letter: PL/CMO(93)4, PL/CNO(93)3).

32. Department of Health. *On the State of the Public Health: the annual report of the Chief Medical Officer for the Department of Health for the year 1992.* London: HMSO, 1993; 130-1.

33. Ekelund H, Finnstrom O, Gunnarskog J, Kallen B, Larsson Y. Administration of vitamin K to newborn infants and childhood cancer. *BMJ* 1993; **307**: 89-91.

34. Klebanoff MA, Read JS, Mills JL, Shiono PH. The risk of childhood cancer after neonatal exposure to vitamin K. *N Engl J Med* 1993; **329:** 905-8.

35. Department of Health. *Neonatal Intensive Care: access to and availability of specialist services: report of a CSAG Working Group.* London: HMSO, 1993. Chair: Professor Sir David Hull.

36. British Paediatric Association. *The Care of Critically Ill Children: report of the multidisciplinary working party on paediatric intensive care convened by the British Paediatric Association.* London: British Paediatric Association, 1993.

37. National Advisory Body on the Confidential Enquiry into Stillbirths and Deaths in Infancy, Department of Health. *Report: March 1992-July 1993.* London: Department of Health, 1993. Chair: Lady Littler.

38. Department of Health. *Services for People with Learning Disabilities and Challenging Behaviour or Mental Health Needs: a report of a project group.* London: HMSO, 1993. Chair: Professor James Mansell.

39. House of Commons. *Health Services for Physically Disabled People aged 16 to 64: 61st Report from the Committee of Public Accounts* (HC 538).

40. National Audit Office. *Health Services for Physically Disabled People Aged 16-64.* London: HMSO, 1992 (HC65).

41. Report of a Working Group convened by the Director of the Public Health Laboratory Service on behalf of the Chief Medical Officer. The incidence and prevalence of AIDS and other severe HIV disease in England and Wales for 1992-7: projections using data to the end of June 1992. *Commun Dis Rep* 1993; **3 (Suppl)**: S1-S17. Chair: Professor Nicholas Day.

42. Department of Health. *AIDS-HIV Infected Health Care Workers: practical guidance on notifying patients. Recommendations of the Expert Advisory Group on AIDS.* Heywood (Lancashire): Department of Health, 1993.

43. Department of Health. *AIDS-HIV Infected Health Care Workers. Guidance on the management of infected health care workers.* Heywood (Lancashire): Department of Health, 1993

44. Department of Health. *Protecting Health Care Workers and Patients from Hepatitis B.* Heywood (Lancashire): Department of Health, 1993 (Health Service Guidelines: HSG(93)40).

45. Department of Health. *Diphtheria in the former USSR.* Heywood (Lancashire): Department of Health, 1993 (Professional Letter: PL(CMO(93)9).

46. Bradley D. Prophylaxis against malaria for travellers from the United Kingdom. *BMJ* 1993; **306:** 1247-52.

47. Department of Health. *Arrangements to deal with health aspects of chemical contamination incidents.* Heywood (Lancashire): Department of Health, 1993 (Health Service Guidelines: HSG(93)38).

48. Department of Health. *Potassium iodate (stable iodine) prophylaxis in the event of a nuclear accident.* Heywood (Lancashire): Department of Health, 1993 (Professional Letter: PL/CMO(93)1).

49. Department of Health. *Nuclear emergency planning in the NHS: distribution of stable iodine (potassium iodate tablets): role of Health Authorities.* Heywood (Lancashire): Department of Health, 1993 (Miscellaneous Circular: 93(50); annex to Health Circular: HC(89)8).

50. Ministry of Agriculture, Fisheries and Food. *Eels: advice to consumers.* London: MAFF, 1993 (Food Safety Directorate News Release: FSD 27/93).

51. Department of Health. *Planning the Medical Workforce: Medical Manpower Standing Advisory Committee: first report.* London: Department of Health, 1993.

52. Department of Health. *Medical and Dental Staffing: part-time consultants.* Heywood (Lancashire): Department of Health, 1993 (Executive Letter: EL(93)39).

53. Department of Health. *Minister endorses measures to tackle shortfall of doctors in 21st century.* London: Department of Health, 1993 (Press Release: H93/710).

54. Department of Health. *Hospital Doctors: training for the future: the report of the Working Group on Specialist Medical Training.* London: Department of Health, 1993.

55. Department of Health. *Undergraduate Medical and Dental Education Research Research: third (interim) report of the Steering Group.* Heywood (Lancashire): Department of Health, 1993.

56. Cochius JI, Mack K, Burns RJ, Alderman CP, Blumbergs PC. Creutzfeldt-Jakob disease in a recipient of human pituitary-derived gonadotrophin. *Aust NZ J Med* 1990; **20**: 592-3.

57. Department of Health. *Creutzfeldt-Jakob disease from treatment with human pituitary gonadotrophin.* Heywood (Lancashire): Department of Health, 1993 (Professional Letter: PL/CMO(93)11).

27

58. Nuffield Council on Bioethics. *Genetic Screening: ethical issues: report of a working party.* London: Nuffield Council on Bioethics, 1993. Chair Professor Dame June Lloyd.

59. Department of Health. *Making London Better.* Heywood (Lancashire): Department of Health, 1993.

60. Department of Health, Department for Education. *Report of the Inquiry into London's Health Service, Medical Education and Research: presented to the Secretaries of State for Health and Education by Sir Bernard Tomlinson.* London: HMSO, 1992.

61. Department of Health. *The Government's Response to the ACOST Report on Medical Research and Health.* London: Department of Health, 1993.

62. Cabinet Office, Advisory Council on Science and Technology. *A Report on Medical Research and Health.* London: HMSO, 1993.

63. Office of Public Service and Science. *Realising Our Potential: a strategy for science, engineering and technology.* London, HMSO, 1993. (Cm. 2250).

64. Department of Health. *Research for Health.* London: Department of Health, 1993.

65. Department of Health. *Fundamental Review of Dental Remuneration: report of Sir Kenneth Bloomfield KCB.* London: Department of Health, 1992.

66. House of Commons, Health Committee. *Dental Services: fourth report from the Health Committee: session 1992-93.* London: HMSO, 1993 (HC 264, vols I-II).

CHAPTER 1

VITAL STATISTICS

(a)   Population size

The estimated resident population of England at 30 June 1993 was 48.5 million, an increase of 154,000 (0.3%) compared with 1992. There was a natural increase (the excess of births over deaths) of 114,000 and net inward migration of 40,000 between mid-1992 and mid-1993.

(b)   Age and sex structure of the resident population

Appendix Table A.1 shows how the sizes of populations in various age-groups have changed in the periods 1981-91, 1991-92 and 1992-93. Although numbers of births fell slightly in each of the two years immediately preceding mid-1993, the number of children below school age (0-4 years) has remained fairly stable. The population of children of school age (5-15 years) is now beginning to increase slowly, after falling during the 1980s. The relatively small late-1970s birth cohorts are now entering the youngest working age-group (16-29 years), the size of which is consequently declining. Larger cohorts born in the period after World War II, up to and including the 1960s, are now in the older working age-groups (30-64 years for men and 30-59 years for women), which are increasing in size. Numbers in the youngest pensioner age-group (65-74 years for men and 60-74 years for women) remain stable. Those aged 75-84 years have fallen slightly in number as survivors from the small cohorts born during World War I reach this age-group, but the most elderly group (aged 85 years and over) continues to grow quite rapidly. Figure 1.1 shows that this most elderly group represents a growing proportion of all pensioners. About two-thirds of persons above pensionable age (65 years for men and 60 years for women), and three-quarters of those aged 85 years and over, are women.

(c)   Fertility statistics - aspects of relevance for health care

Total conceptions

Data on conceptions relate to pregnancies which led to a maternity or to a legal termination under the Abortion Act 1967[1,2]; they exclude spontaneous and illegal abortions. The redevelopment of computer systems has resulted in delays to some births and abortions data. The latest available conceptions data are for 1991, when 808,989 conceptions occurred to women resident in England, a fall on the 1990 figure. The overall conception rate in 1991 was 77.8 per 1,000 women aged 15-44 years (this figure differs from that quoted in last year's Report because of re-based population data).

29

Figure 1.1: *Population aged 60/65-74 years, 75-84 years and 85 years and over, England, 1981-93*

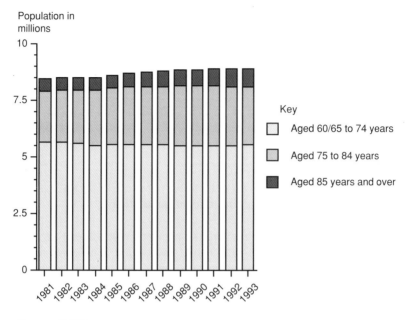

Source: OPCS

Total births

The number of birth registrations has been used to produce an estimate of 674,000 live births in England and Wales during 1993; births in England typically account for 95% of the combined England and Wales figure. There were estimated to be 640,000 live births in England in 1993, 2% lower than in 1992. In 1992, there were 651,784 live births, of which 31% occurred outside marriage.

Fertility in women of 30 years-of-age and over

During 1992, the fertility rate of women in their early 30s exceeded that of women in their early 20s for the first time since data were collected. Furthermore, the fertility of women in their late 30s was greater than that of teenagers. These figures indicate a change in the timing of childbearing over the past decade. As cohorts of women born after 1945 have progressively delayed childbearing, so the fertility rates have fallen at younger ages and risen at older ages. A fall of 4% in fertility occurred to women aged 20-24 years between 1991 and 1992. The fertility rate of women in their early 30s has remained fairly constant over the past 3 years (see Figure 1.2), after a rise of 27% in the previous decade. The fertility rate for women in their late 30s continued to rise (by 4%

Figure 1.2: *Percentage change in fertility rates by age-group, England, 1982-92 (1982 = 100%)*

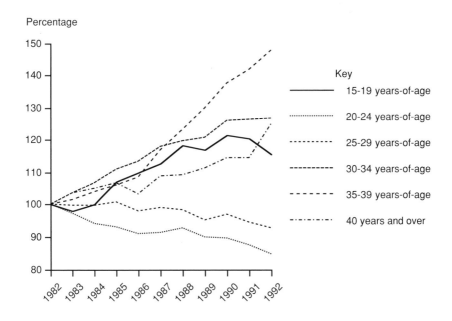

Source: OPCS

between 1991 and 1992), to reach its highest level since the previous peak in 1970. The rate for women aged 40 years and over also rose, to 5.9 births per 1,000 women in 1992, over 9% higher than in the previous year and continuing the steady increase seen over the past decade. However, this rate was still lower than the 1972 rate of 7.7 births per 1,000 women aged over 40 years.

The trend of delayed childbearing has also resulted in a rise in childlessness at each age-group among women born since 1945 (see Figure 1.3). Over a third of women born in 1960 reached 30 years-of-age without having had a child - twice the equivalent proportion for women born in 1945. Permanent childlessness has also risen and contributed to a fall in average completed family size. The increased fertility of women aged over 30 years is unlikely to reverse this fall.

Teenage conceptions in 1991

The number and rate of conceptions among older teenagers aged 15-19 years have fallen in 1991, after rising since 1983 (see Figure 1.4). The overall conception rate fell by 6% between 1990 and 1991. A third of all conceptions to teenagers led to an abortion, although this proportion also fell slightly between 1990 and 1991.

Figure 1.3: *Percentage of women childless at successive ages, cohorts born in 1945, 1950, 1955, 1960 and 1965, England and Wales*

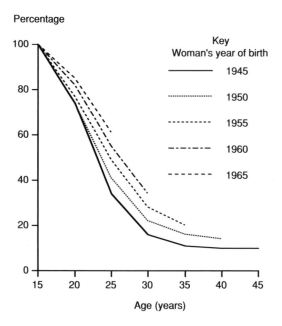

Source: OPCS

For girls aged under 16 years, the rate of conception leading to a maternity rose by around 50% over the decade, although just over half of all conceptions end in abortion. (see Figure 1.5).

Regional variations in conception rates are examined in Table 1.1. The rates of conception for all teenagers were greatest in more urban areas. For girls aged less than 16 years, the highest overall rates occurred in the 'principal cities', with 13.3 conceptions per 1,000 women compared with rates of 9.3 per 1,000 for England as a whole, and of 5.7 per 1,000 in 'mixed urban-rural' areas (which have the lowest rate). Inner London showed the highest rate of conceptions leading to an abortion for all teenagers.

Abortions

Based on provisional data, a total of 150,802 abortions were performed in 1993 under the Abortion Act 1967[1,2] on women who were resident in England. This represents a decrease of 2,837 (2%) compared with 1992, but an increase of 29,291 (24%) compared with 1983. Of the total, 89% were carried out at under 13 weeks gestation, and only 3% were performed beyond 16 weeks gestation.

In 1993, 30% of all abortions carried out on resident women were on those in their early 20s, whilst only 12% were on those aged 35 years and over. The abortion rate was highest among women aged 20-24 years (25.7 abortions per 1,000 women aged 20-24 years).

Figure 1.4: *Conception rates by outcome for females aged 15-19 years, England, 1971-91*

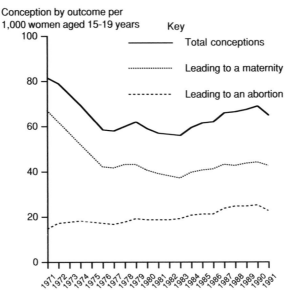

Note: Data for 1973 are unavailable.

Source: OPCS

Figure 1.5: *Conception rates by outcome for females aged under 16 years, England, 1971-91*

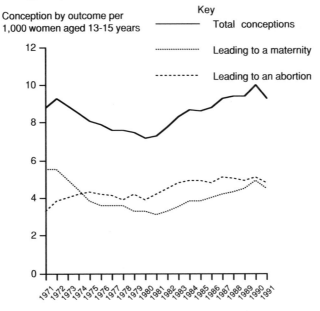

Notes: Data for 1973 are unavailable.
        The vertical scale differs from that used in Figure 1.4.

Source: OPCS

Table 1.1: Conception rates for women aged under 20 years by area aggregates*, England, 1991

Area	Rates per 1000 women aged 13-15 years			Rates per 1000 women aged 15-19 years		
	All conceptions	Leading to maternities	Leading to abortions	All conceptions	Leading to maternities	Leading to abortions
England	9.3	4.5	4.8	64.8	42.2	22.6
(Number)	(7368)	(3593)	(3775)	(96866)	(63134)	(33732)
Greater London	9.0	4.2	4.8	70.8	39.7	31.2
Inner London	12.5	6.3	6.2	90.4	51.1	39.3
Outer London	7.2	3.2	4.0	59.9	33.3	26.6
Metropolitan districts	12.5	6.8	5.8	80.3	56.6	23.7
Principal cities	13.3	7.5	5.8	83.2	58.4	24.8
Others	12.2	6.5	5.7	79.1	55.9	23.2
Non-metropolitan districts	8.2	3.8	4.4	57.7	37.3	20.4
Cities	12.7	7.0	5.7	77.1	54.1	23.1
Industrial	10.5	5.2	5.3	70.7	48.8	22.0
With new towns	10.4	5.1	5.3	71.2	49.0	22.2
Resort and retirement	7.9	3.6	4.3	58.4	37.5	21.0
Mixed urban-rural	5.7	2.2	3.5	43.5	24.5	19.0
Remoter larger rural	6.3	2.5	3.8	47.9	30.1	17.8

* Described in Appendix 5 of *Key Population and Vital Statistics: local and health authority area, 1991*. London: HMSO, 1993 (Series VS no. 18) .

Source: OPCS

In 1993, 18% of legal abortions were on women aged under 20 years; of these, 11% were on girls aged under 16 years. Over the past decade, abortions on women aged under 20 years have risen from 14.9 per 1,000 women aged 14-19 years in 1983 to 16.5 per 1,000 in 1993.

References

1.   *Abortion Act 1967.* London: HMSO, 1967.
2.   *Abortion Act 1967 (as amended by Statutory Instrument SI 480c. 10).* London: HMSO, 1991.

(d)   Mortality

The estimated number of deaths registered in England during 1993 was 544,000. The estimated crude mortality rate increased from 10.8 per 1,000 population in 1992, to 11.1 per 1,000 in 1993.

Influenza

Although little detail is yet available for mortality figures in 1993, the Registrar General's Weekly Return was prepared clerically and published as usual; it includes the total number of deaths registered each week, and deaths from some infectious diseases, as well as cases of some infectious diseases reported by a sample of general practitioners (GPs).

The total number of deaths in October was higher than normally expected. The expected number of deaths is calculated by taking a 10-year average of the number of deaths in corresponding weeks, and adjusting to allow for trends in deaths and in the age structure of the population[1]. Cases of epidemic influenza and influenza-like illnesses in general practice were also increasing rapidly.

During the last major influenza outbreak in 1989/90, only 10% of the 'excess' deaths (those observed minus those expected) were ascribed to influenza infection[2], although another 20% were certified with pneumonia as the underlying cause. Thus the total numbers of deaths, deaths from pneumonia and influenza deaths were monitored.

Appendix Figure A.1 shows that the total number of deaths registered was high between early October (week 40) and the end of the year. However, the number of deaths was much lower than in the last major outbreak of influenza, which peaked at over 18,000 deaths in one week. The maximum number of deaths (week 48, in early December) was about 14,000, which was more than 2,000 higher than the expected number of deaths. This maximum occurred about one month earlier than in 1989/90.

The maximum number of deaths in a week with influenza given as the underlying cause was 60 in the week ending 10 December (week 49); notifications of influenza infection peaked rather earlier, in the week ending 14 November, with a notification rate of over 230 cases per 100,000 population.

Figure 1.6 compares the notification rates of influenza and influenza-like illnesses in 1993-94 with data from the last major outbreak in 1989-90, and with an average of the three intervening years (1990-91 to 1992-93) in which there were no influenza outbreaks. By comparison to 1989-90, the peak was much lower and occurred earlier in the year.

Figure 1.6: *Notification rates of influenza and influenza-like illnesses, England and Wales, 1989-90 to 1993-94*

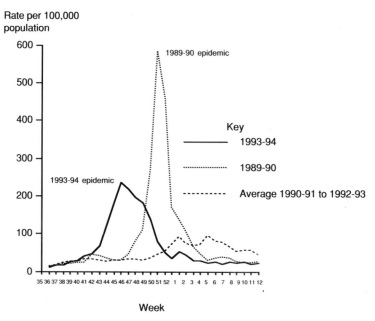

Source: Weekly Returns Service, RCGP, Birmingham

The total number of deaths from influenza was small; over 80% were among those aged 75 years and over, and 50% in those aged 85 years and over. No age breakdown is available yet for excess deaths where influenza was not given as the underlying cause.

Suicide and undetermined deaths

The Report for 1992 included data on suicide trends and regional variations. Figure 1.7 shows the methods used to commit suicide by men and women, respectively. Until the 1960s, when natural gas was introduced, poisoning by domestic gases was the most common method used to commit suicide for men and women alike. Over recent years, the number of deaths among men from poisoning by other gases (mostly carbon monoxide from motor vehicle exhausts) has increased rapidly, now accounting for over a quarter of suicides. Among women, nearly half of all suicides are caused by poisoning.

36

Figure 1.7: *Suicides and undetermined deaths, England and Wales, 1988-92*

Males

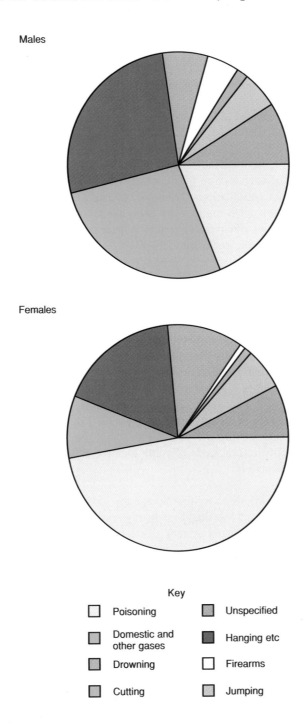

Females

Key

☐	Poisoning	▨	Unspecified
▨	Domestic and other gases	■	Hanging etc
▨	Drowning	☐	Firearms
▨	Cutting	▨	Jumping

Source: OPCS

References

1. Bulusu L. Monitoring weekly deaths. *Population Trends* 1983; **34:** 20-5.
2. Ashley J, Smith T, Dunnell K. Deaths in Great Britain associated with the influenza epidemic of 1989/90.
    Population Trends 1991; **65:** 16-20.

(e)   Prevalence of disease in the community

Morbidity statistics from general practice

Between 1 September 1991 and 31 August 1992, 60 general practices in England
and Wales took part in the fourth of a series of studies of GPs and their patients
(MSGP-4). Details of each face-to-face contact with a patient were recorded,
including the reason for consultation. Demographic data were collected from all
patients on the practices' NHS registers by interview. The population covered
was nearly half a million. Preliminary results will be published early in 1994,
with a fuller account available in Autumn 1994.

During that year, 78% of people consulted a health care professional in general
practice at least once. For the rest of this section, the proportion consulting will
mean the proportion per 10,000 of a particular group who consulted for a
particular condition at least once during the year. Highest proportions consulting
were among children aged under 5 years; this proportion fell among those aged
5-44 years, but then increased with advancing age. Differences by age and
severity of disease or condition are shown in Figure 1.8.

Diseases and conditions were classified according to the 9th revision of the
International Classification of Diseases (ICD). Figure 1.9 shows the proportions
consulting at least once during the year for each chapter of the ICD. The
supplementary classification includes consultations for other reasons, such as
vaccination and contraception.

Figure 1.10 shows proportions consulting by age for some of the main chapters
of the ICD. For children aged less than 5 years, high proportions consulting were
seen for diseases of the respiratory system, diseases of the nervous system and
sense organs, and infectious diseases (65%, 43% and 36%, respectively). This
pattern was similar in older children, although proportions consulting were much
lower.

Among those aged 16-44 years, the proportions consulting were generally low.
For many diseases these proportions increased steadily beyond the age of 45
years, particularly for circulatory diseases, digestive diseases, mental disorders,
musculoskeletal diseases, and cancers. The proportions consulting for almost all
conditions were high among elderly people.

Table 1.2 shows proportions consulting for various diseases: for diseases
confined to females, rates of 29 per 10,000 were reported for malignant neoplasm
of the breast, 4 per 10,000 for malignant neoplasm of the cervix, and 206 per

Figure 1.8: *Severity of disease or condition among patients consulting in general practice, England and Wales, 1991-92*

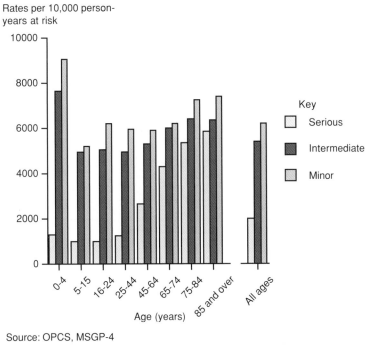

Source: OPCS, MSGP-4

Figure 1.9: *Classification of disease or condition among patients consulting in general practice, England and Wales, 1991-92*

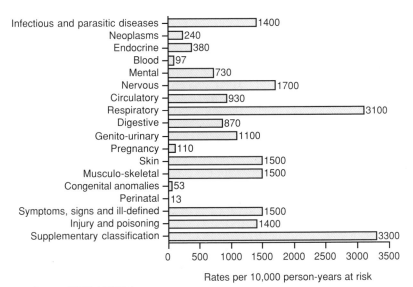

Source: OPCS, MSGP-4

Figure 1.10: *Proportions of patients consulting in general practice by age-group and disease category, England and Wales, 1991-92*

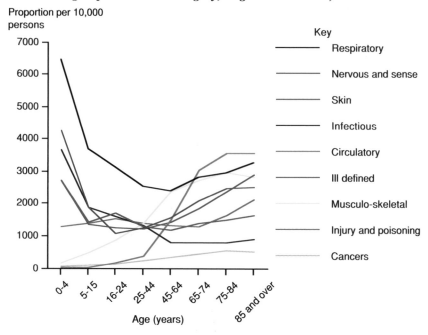

Source: OPCS, MSGP-4

Table 1.2: *Consultation rates in general practice for various diseases, England and Wales, 1991-92*

Disease	Consultation rates per 10,000 person-years at risk
Malignant neoplasm of trachea, bronchus and lung	7
Melanoma of the skin	2
Other malignant neoplasm of the skin	7
Diabetes mellitus	111
Disorders of lipid metabolism	61
Obesity	82
Neurotic disorders	344
Alcohol dependence	13
Drug dependence	19
Acute reaction to stress	26
Depressive disorders not elsewhere classified	110
Migraine	115
Essential hypertension	412
Ischaemic heart disease	170
Cerebrovascular disorders	66
Asthma	425
Contact dermatitis and eczema	203
Psoriasis and similar disorders	73

Source: OPCS, MSGP-4

Figure 1.11: *Three-year moving averages of measures of morbidity from the General Household Survey, males and females, Great Britain, 1979-92*

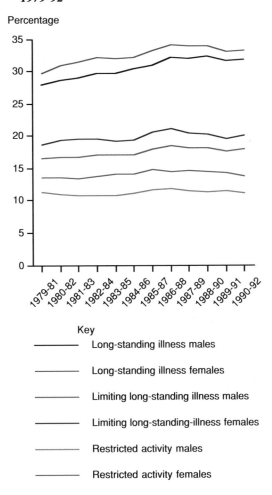

Percentage

Key

——————— Long-standing illness males

——————— Long-standing illness females

——————— Limiting long-standing illness males

——————— Limiting long-standing-illness females

——————— Restricted activity males

——————— Restricted activity females

Source: OPCS, GHS

10,000 for inflammatory diseases of the pelvic organs; for diseases confined to males, a rate of 12 per 10,000 was reported for malignant neoplasm of the prostate.

Chronic sickness

The General Household Survey (GHS)[1] is a continuous survey collecting information about 20,000 adults and 5,000 children in Great Britain each year. It provides two measures of chronic sickness. Firstly, people are asked whether they have any long-standing illness, disability or infirmity. Those who answer yes are then asked "What is the matter with you?", and then whether this limits their activities in any way. Acute sickness is measured by asking whether, in the two weeks before interview, people had to cut down on any of the things they

41

usually do because of illness or injury. In 1992, 32% reported a long-standing illness, 19% a limiting long-standing illness and 12% restricted activity in the previous two weeks. Figure 1.11 shows trends from 1979 to 1992 for these three measures for males and females separately. The data are presented as three-year moving averages to smooth out year-on-year fluctuations. The prevalence of acute sickness has changed little. The prevalence of reported long-standing illness increased during the 1980s; towards the end of the decade the increase slowed, and then a slight fall occurred.

A question on long-term illness was also asked in the 1991 Census. An analysis of the results of this question in Great Britain will be published early in 1994[2]. However, the proportions of the population with a limiting long-term illness appear to vary among different ethnic groups, even when age-standardised to allow for different age structures.

Health Survey data

The type of condition reported as the cause of long-standing illness was analysed by ICD group in the 1989 GHS, and also in the 1991 Health Survey for England[3]. Illnesses associated with the musculo-skeletal system were most frequently mentioned as the cause of long-standing illness, followed by the heart and circulatory system and the respiratory system.

References

1. Office of Population Censuses and Surveys. *General Household Survey 1991*. London: HMSO, 1993 (Series GHS no. 20).
2. Office of Population Censuses and Surveys. *1991 Census: limiting long-term illness, Great Britain*. London: HMSO, 1993.
3. Office of Population Censuses and Surveys. *Health Survey for England 1991*. London: HMSO, 1993.

(f)   Infant and perinatal mortality

Due to re-development of computer systems, no reliable figures for infant or perinatal mortality for 1993 are yet available. However, between 1991 and 1992 the infant mortality rate in England fell for babies of mothers of all ages. The greatest fall (of 19%) occurred among women aged under 20 years. For babies born inside marriage in 1992, the infant mortality rate was 31% lower than for babies born outside marriage. Between 1991 and 1992, the infant mortality rate for babies born within marriage fell by 10%, compared with a fall of 13% for babies born outside marriage.

During 1992 in England, 49% of all liveborn babies with a stated birthweight who died in the first six days of life weighed under 1,500 grams at birth, although only 1% of live births were below this weight. Between 1991 and 1992, the post-neonatal mortality rate (deaths between 28 days and 1 year of age) fell by 33% among babies who weighed 3,000 grams or more at birth, but by only 2% among babies who weighed under 1,500 grams at birth.

(g)   Trends in cancer* incidence and mortality

Data from the 1988 and 1989 GHS show that 1% of adults reported cancer as a cause of long-standing illness. This estimate can be compared with that based on the Office of Population Censuses and Surveys (OPCS) Longitudinal Study, which is discussed in the report of the 1990 review of the cancer registration system[1]. The study brings together, for 1% of the population, information from the National Cancer Registration Scheme, successive censuses and death registration. It suggests that just over half a million people alive in 1981 would have had a cancer registered in the preceding ten years - again a prevalence of around 1%.

The latest national totals of cancer registrations relate to 1989. Appendix Tables A.7 and A.8 show the numbers registered by age, sex and site. Although trends over the period 1979-89 must be interpreted with caution, for all malignant neoplasms (excluding non-melanoma skin cancer) there was an increase of over 10%. When specific sites of malignancy are examined there are some trends of note.

When adjusted for age, lung cancer registration decreased for males but increased for females between 1979 and 1989. For both sexes there were large increases in the number of registrations of malignant melanoma of the skin during the period 1979-89. During the same period there was a decrease in registrations of stomach cancer. There were marked downward trends for lymphosarcoma and reticulosarcoma and for Hodgkin's disease, but an upward trend for other malignant neoplasms of lymphoid and histiocytic tissue, to which less well specified lymphomas would be coded.

There have been upward trends for bladder cancer and malignant neoplasm of the kidney and other unspecified urinary organs between 1979 and 1989. The number of registrations of carcinoma-in-situ of the cervix uteri was very much higher in 1984 than in previous years, and has continued to increase markedly: in 1989, the total number of registrations was approximately double that in 1979. However, in respect of carcinoma-in-situ, possible improvements in the level of completeness of registration and in ascertainment need to be taken into account.

As with the incidence of all cancers, there has been no decline in mortality in recent years. Age-standardised death rates since the 1920s were shown in last year's Report[2]. For males, the post-war rise levelled off in the 1970s. For females, there was a declining trend until the early 1960s, followed by a rise. Within these totals, however, there was a rise and then a fall in the rate for cancer of the lung/bronchus in males, contrasting with a continuing rise in females. There was a steady fall in the rate for cancer of the stomach in both sexes.

* cancer = malignant neoplasm

References

1.   Office of Population Censuses and Surveys. *Review of the National cancer registration system: report of the Working Group of the Registrar General's Medical Advisory Committee.* London: HMSO, 1990 (Series MB1 no. 17).

2. Department of Health. *On the State of the Public Health: the annual report of the Chief Medical Officer of the Department of Health for the year 1992*. London: HMSO, 1993; 44.

(h)   Trends in reporting congenital malformations

Appendix Table A.6 shows that, according to provisional data for 1993, the number of malformed live births in England decreased to 5,292, 6% lower than in 1992.

(i)   Appendix Tables and their content (pages 203-213)

Appendix Table 1: *Population age and sex structure, England, 1993, and changes by age, 1981-92 and 1992-93.*

This table is described on the first page of this chapter.

Appendix Table 2: *Five main causes of death for males and females at different ages, England 1992.*

This table contrasts the major causes of mortality in different age-groups. It is reproduced from last year's Report[1] because OPCS data for 1993 are not available.

Appendix Table 3: *Relative mortality from various conditions when presented as numbers of deaths and future years of 'working life' lost, England and Wales, 1992.*

This table is reproduced from last year's Report[2] because OPCS data for 1993 are not available.

Appendix Table 4: *Trends in 'avoidable' deaths, England and Wales, 1979-92.*

This table is reproduced from last year's Report[3] because OPCS data for 1993 are not available.

Appendix Table 5: *Live births, stillbirths, infant mortality and abortions, England, 1960-93.*

Trends are discussed in this chapter.

Appendix Table 6: *Congenital malformations - trends in selected malformations, England, 1980, 1985, 1992 and 1993.*

Trends are noted in this chapter.

Appendix Table 7: *Cancer registration, England and Wales, 1989 (males).*

The table indicates the distribution of cancer registrations in men at different ages. At all ages combined, cancers of the lung, large intestine (including rectum) and prostate account for about half of the registrations. In childhood, a high proportion of cancers are attributable to leukaemias, lymphomas, tumours of the central nervous system, and embryonic tumours such as neuroblastomas and retinoblastomas. At older ages, cancer of the lung is the major cause registered. In the oldest age-group presented (85 years and over), prostate cancer accounts for slightly more registrations than lung cancer.

Appendix Table 8: *Cancer registrations, England and Wales, 1989 (females).*

In childhood, the pattern of female cancers is broadly similar to that in males. However, in the 25-44 years age-group cancers of the breast (41%) and cervix (17%) predominate. At older ages, breast cancer continues to account for many registrations, although cancers of the lung, skin and large intestine also occur in substantial numbers.

Appendix Table 9: *Immunisation uptake, England, 1980-92/93.*

The information presented in this table is discussed in Chapter 6 (see page 154).

Appendix Table 10: *Cumulative total of AIDS cases by exposure category, England, to 31 December 1993.*

Recent trends in AIDS cases are discussed in Chapter 6 (see page 141).

Appendix Figure 1: *Weekly deaths, England and Wales, 1992 and 1993, and expected deaths, 1993.*

This figure illustrates the week-by-week registrations of deaths from all causes at ages one year and over for 1992 and 1993. These can be compared with the expected values for 1993 based on an average of deaths registered in the same week in the previous ten years, adjusted to allow for trends in death rates and in population.

References

1. Department of Health. *On the State of the Public Health: the annual report of the Chief Medical Officer of the Department of Health for the year 1992.* London: HMSO, 1993; 46, 212.
2. Department of Health. *On the State of the Public Health. the annual report of the Chief Medical Officer of the Department of Health for the year 1992.* London, HMSO, 1993; 46, 213.
3. Department of Health. *On the State of the Public Health: the annual report of the Chief Medical Officer of the Department of Health for the year 1992.* London, HMSO, 1993; 47, 214.

CHAPTER 2

THE NATION'S HEALTH

(a)   Public health in England

The Public Health Network

In 1992, the first steps were taken to develop a national Public Health Network to draw together public health skills and specialist knowledge to support the improvement of the public health[1]. During 1993, the central network met four times and discussed a wide range of public health issues of relevance to the Department of Health (DH) and to public health practitioners in the National Health Service (NHS); a need for specialist groups in communicable disease control and health promotion was identified and these groups are being established.

A major aim of the network is to improve communication, and it soon became apparent that there was a need for improved means to ensure rapid transfer of information within the medical profession whenever there was a threat to the public health which required widespread urgent action. As a first step an electronic networking system (EPINET) between District Directors of Public Health (DDsPH), was set up, supplemented by locally arranged cascade systems, and will be available for use from Spring 1994.

Surveillance of the public health function

For the last three years, DH has examined the progress made towards implementation of the Health Circular HC(88)64[2], *Health of the Population: responsibilities of Health Authorities*, and to determine the impact of the National Health Service and Community Care Act 1990[3] and the strategy for health[4] on the public health function. This surveillance programme continued during 1993, with a series of informal visits made to Regional Directors of Public Health (RDsPH), heads of academic departments of public health and Regional General Mangers (RGMs).

The results from a national questionnaire survey of DDsPH undertaken by North West Thames Regional Health Authority (RHA) showed that, in 1991, the requirements of HC(88)64 in terms of Director of Public Health (DPH) appointments and the production of annual reports were almost universally met. The 1993 survey showed that the DPH annual reports mostly influenced service expansion, new working arrangements or commissioning of research. In 1991, 20% of DsPH were the chief source of public health advice to other agencies; by 1993, this figure had increased to 98%. Similarly, advice to Family Health Services Authorities (FHSAs) by departments of public health medicine rose from 41% in 1991 to 76% in 1993. Virtually all respondents (92% in 1991, 96% in 1993) were assessing health needs for DHAs, including consultation with local communities.

Abrams Committee

Changes in the organisation and management of the NHS have meant that the mechanisms by which the NHS maintains its important public health function have required review, as indicated in last year's Report[1]. A working party, established in 1992 under the chairmanship of Dr Michael Abrams, formerly Deputy Chief Medical Officer, was given the remit to develop new guidance to assist the NHS in discharging its public health responsibilities; the Committee's advice on public health responsibilities of the NHS, and roles of others (HSG(93)56)[5], was issued on 24 November 1993. This guidance from the Departments of Health and the Environment replaces HC(88)64[2] and EL(91)123[6].

The Committee confirmed the principles outlined in the 1988 report *Public Health in England*[7] and restated the NHS's responsibility for the public health of the population; it emphasised the need for all authorities and agencies to work within a co-ordinated and comprehensive public health strategy, including arrangements for the control of communicable disease and infection and for dealing with the health aspects of non-communicable environmental hazards. DHAs and DDsPH should provide the focus for this co-ordinated strategy.

Communicable disease control

Legislation to update the Public Health (Control of Disease) Act 1984[8] will be brought forward when Parliamentary time allows. Meanwhile, the advice of the Abrams Committee in HSG(93)56[5] incorporates guidance on communicable disease control in an expanded version of EL(91)123[6]. It describes the role of Consultants in Communicable Disease Control (CsCDC) within departments of public health in DHAs, and stresses the need for adequate staffing and support for communicable disease control.

New guidance was given on collaboration between CsCDC and Infection Control Doctors (ICDs) in the management of hospital infection. The lead role in the management of major outbreaks in hospitals may now be taken by the ICDs when the infection involved has no implications for the community. FHSAs, in consultation with District Infection Control Committees, have been asked to ensure that advice on infection control in surgeries is available to all general practitioners (GPs). Local contracts should ensure that relevant laboratory results are rapidly passed on to CsCDC and the Communicable Disease Surveillance Centre (CDSC) of the Public Health Laboratory Service (PHLS).

Funding for public health training

DH continued to support training posts as part of a programme which started in

1988; this scheme has so far trained 154 extra specialists in public health medicine and 10 extra posts were funded for the year 1993/94. DH also funded the Public Health Legal Information Unit, based at Central Manchester Health Authority, to help to improve CsCDC's and environmental health officers' knowledge and understanding of the legal framework under which they work. By the end of the project in July 1994, training courses will have been provided across the country and a comprehensive reference document will be sent to all CsCDC and environmental health departments.

In June 1993, DH funded and organised a third 2-day national conference for CsCDC and planned a fourth conference for October 1994.

The role of nursing professions in public health

During 1993, the Statutory Nursing and Midwifery Professional Advisory Committee (SNMAC) began to examine the contribution that nurses, midwives and health visitors could bring to improving the health of populations.

References

1. Department of Health. *On the State of the Public Health: the annual report of the Chief Medical Officer of the Department of Health for the year 1992.* London: HMSO, 1993: 49-51.
2. Department of Health. *Health Services Management: health of the population: responsibilities of Health Authorities.* Heywood (Lancashire): Department of Health, 1988 (Health Circular: HC(88)64).
3. *National Health Service and Community Care Act 1990.* Lonodn: HMSO, 1990.
4. Department of Health. *The Health of the Nation: a strategy for health in England.* London: HMSO, 1992 (Cm. 1986).
5. Department of Health. Department of Environment. *Public Health: responsibilities of the NHS and roles of others.* Heywood (Lancashire) Department of Health, 1993 (Miscellaneous Circular: MISC(93)56).
6. Department of Health. *Communicable disease control.* London: Department of Health, 1991 (Executive Letter: EL(91)123).
7. *Public Health in England: The Report of the Committee of Inquiry into Future Development of the Public Health Function.* London: HMSO, 1988 (Cm. 289). Chair: Sir Donald Acheson.
8. *Public Health (Control of Disease) Act 1984.* London: HMSO, 1984.

(b)   Regional perspectives

Mersey

The imminent merger with North Western and part of Northern RHAs meant that 1993 was the final year for which a Mersey Regional Public Health Annual Report could be produced. In *The Changing Health of Mersey 1948-1994*[1], the RDPH took the opportunity to review the development of health services during this period, and in particular the role of the RHA. There have been enormous changes in the health needs of the population during this period, but in many ways the configuration of services still lags behind. The present radical approach to implementing a health strategy for the Region reflects the commitment to matching contemporary needs with appropriate responses ranging from health promotion, through primary care and highly specialised treatment, to care in the community.

A review of the annual reports of the Liverpool Regional Hospital Board (1947-1973) showed that, although the Board was mainly interested in hospital matters, many of the issues of concern then are still with us today. For example, the mortality rate in Mersey from tuberculosis fell from 28 per 100,000 in 1952 to three per 100,000 in 1969. This was partly due to improved clinical facilities and the success of a Region-wide mass radiography campaign in the late 1950s. The gradual disappearance of tuberculosis meant that the disease was no longer considered in the Region's annual reports after 1970. However, it shows that the Board had to operate flexibly with regard to the prevailing public health agendas of the day. This responsibility towards the Region's population remains, since it has recently become apparent that tuberculosis can no longer be considered a disease of the past[2]. A contemporary parallel example might be drawn with HIV/AIDS. Although Mersey has a disproportionately high number of intravenous drug misusers, innovations, such as the first full-scale needle-and-syringe exchange scheme in the country, have helped to ensure that transmission of HIV infection among this high-risk group is low.

Mental illness remains a priority. In 1952, there were about 5,000 psychiatric beds available, but hospitals in the Region were in fact catering for 6,000-7,000 patients. However, during the late 1950s and early 1960s, several psychiatric day hospitals were created. This represented a beginning in the shift away from the institutionalisation of the Region's mentally ill patients. Now there are only 514 long-stay beds, whilst health authorities are supporting 'Care in the Community' schemes for over 1,100 people.

In 1948, the annual infant mortality rate in Mersey stood at 49 per 1,000 live births, much higher than the national figure of 35 per 1,000. By the 1990s, the Region's rate had fallen to around seven per 1,000 live births - comparable to, and sometimes below, the national rate. This represents a remarkable reduction in inequality. The emphasis must now be to ensure that the Region's infants remain healthy well into childhood and beyond. The problems children face - such as family breakdown - are very different from those of 1948 and raise fundamental questions about the most appropriate shape of a future child health service. Recognising this, Mersey published a strategy for healthy children[3], which highlighted the need for better information on the socio-economic and demographic characteristics of the Region's child population; more research on which lifestyle factors have the greatest effect on their health; and a greater understanding of the use of health services by children. In common with many other areas of health care, the strategy emphasises the need to change the focus for children from the acute sector to primary care.

Over the last half century, immense changes have taken place in family life and social institutions, patterns of health and disease, and the technologies and interventions which can affect the human condition. These changes make it difficult to see how a commentator writing in 1948 could have anticipated the changes in public health that would take place before the end of the century. It remains to be seen how great the changes will be in the next 46 years.

Oxford

National data on smoking in teenagers in England from the Schools Health Education Unit at the University of Exeter provide information on 29,074 young people aged 11-16 years[4]. The results indicate that by the age of 16 years, one-third of teenagers will never have smoked cigarettes, one-third will have tried and given up and one-third will be smoking either regularly or occasionally.

To try to prevent teenagers from becoming regular smokers, and to obtain local data on smoking rates comparable to those collected nationally, 18 upper schools in four counties - Oxfordshire, Northamptonshire, Berkshire and Buckinghamshire - will participate in a programme to assess the effectiveness of feeding back information about individual health risk behaviours to individual teenagers.

All pupils of 12 schools who are in their 9th year of schooling (aged 12-14 years) will be asked to complete a questionnaire that includes details about their smoking habits. In six schools the results of the questionnaire will be analysed to give individual risk scores for discussion with each child; in the other six schools, only general information about overall health behaviours of pupils will be fed back. Two years later, all pupils in the 11th year of schooling in the original 12 schools, and similar pupils in a further six schools will again be questioned about health behaviour. Data will be analysed to see whether there are any significant differences between the smoking rates and other health behaviours among the pupils in the three different sets of schools.

Another fruitful and developing area of smoking cessation intervention is the use of peer group education. The 'Stub it Club', based at Manor School in Northampton, was begun in 1990 and uses young people to get across facts about smoking to their peers and to encourage them to stop. Further initiatives are being developed in the Region, including investigation of the ways in which primary health care can best adapt itself to help teenagers who are smoking and who want to give up.

Northern

In last year's Report[5], the Chief Medical Officer drew attention to the importance of action to ensure that the care delivered by doctors and other health care professionals is as effective as possible. Clinical effectiveness is an issue which is being addressed by the medical profession in individual hospitals and general practices, as well as at national level through the Royal Colleges and other professional bodies. It is also an issue for all Health Authorities that purchase health care for the populations for which they are responsible.

In the Northern Region, this theme was emphasised in response to the priority given to it by the Chief Medical Officer. The RDPH's introduction to his report[6] points out that if more women who were expected to have premature babies were given a short course of corticosteroid, which is cheap and simple to administer, then fewer such babies would die and fewer would be born with lung impairment. This benefit was demonstrated in research carried out more than 20 years ago[7], but has not yet entered mainstream health practice. For example, in the Northern Region, of the mothers with babies born before 32 weeks' gestation in 1990 and 1991, only one in eight had received steroids in labour, and maternity units differed greatly in the extent to which steroids were used; the position has now improved after managers and health care professionals reviewed local policies.

There are many similar issues: widespread adoption of properly validated research will improve the quality of patient care. Similarly, treatments which are ineffective are not worth using: the revenues saved could be spent on providing effective health interventions.

The Northern Region has identified seven areas for particular attention:

- to ensure that more patients with hypertension get the appropriate treatment to reduce the incidence of heart attacks and strokes;

- to encourage GPs to prescribe generically ten common medicines, which should save £2.6 million with no reduction in quality of care;

- to raise the proportion of day-care operations;

- to emphasise the need for early antibiotic treatment in children suspected to have meningococcal meningitis;

- to prevent tooth decay by the introduction of fluoridation to water supplies; *and*

- to raise the quality of life of mentally ill people by improving their housing.

The RDPH for the Northern Region, following the Chief Medical Officer's lead, framed his report as a series of challenges. Why don't we change our way of treating patients in line with the latest research? Why don't we introduce public health measures known to be of benefit to the population? These questions have stimulated debate and discussion throughout the Region and among local media and patient groups. Highlighting of such issues and any scope for improvement will help to ensure that the quality of health care can be made even better.

References

1. Mersey Regional Health Authority. *The Changing Health of Mersey 1948-1994*. Liverpool: Mersey Regional Health Authority (in press).
2. Spence DPS, Hotchkiss J, Williams CSD, Davies PDO. Tuberculosis and poverty. *BMJ* 1993; **307**: 759-61.
3. Mersey Regional Health Authority. *A strategy for healthy children*. Liverpool: Mersey Regional Health Authority, 1993.
4. Balding J. *Young people in 1993*. Exeter: University of Exeter School of Education, 1993.
5. Department of Health. *On the State of the Public Health: the annual report of the Chief Medical Officer of the Department of Health for the year 1992*. London: HMSO; 1993: 107-10.
6. Northern Regional Health Authority. *Health Report*. Newcastle-upon-Tyne: Northern Regional Health Authority, 1993.
7. Liggins GC, Howie RN. A controlled trial of antepartum corticosteroid treatment for prevention of the respiratory distress syndrome in premature infants. *Paediatrics* 1972; **50**: 515-25.

(c)   Inter-Departmental Group on Public Health

The Inter-Departmental Group on Public Health, chaired by the Chief Medical Officer, facilitates inter-Departmental discussion and exchange of information on health issues. The Group usually meets three times a year and is intended: to keep under review hazards to public health; to provide advice to Government on the assessment of such hazards; to provide an Inter-Departmental forum for the discussion of scientific or technical issues that bear on public health; and to strengthen and to support existing links between other Government Departments and to identify and to correct any gaps in communications.

The composition of the Group reflects public health interests across Government departments. It includes representatives from the Cabinet Office, DH, the Ministry of Agriculture, Fisheries and Food, the Department of the Environment, the Home Office, the Foreign and Commonwealth Office, the Ministry of Defence, the Department of Social Security, the Department of Health and Social Services for Northern Ireland, the Scottish Office Home and Health Department, the Welsh Office, the Department of Transport, the Office of Public Service and Science and the Health and Safety Executive.

(d)   Sickness at work

Avoidable ill-health is an expensive burden - and not just to the health service. The direct cost to industry of sickness absences in the United Kingdom (UK) was recently estimated to be £13 billion annually[1]. Eight million days annually are lost through alcohol and drink-related disease and 80 million days are lost through mental illness, at an estimated cost of over £5 billion. An additional 50 million days are lost in the UK because of smoking-related diseases. Efforts to reduce avoidable ill-health will therefore benefit employers as well as employees.

The impact of actions to reduce ill-health at work can only be assessed if effective and accurate procedures are in place to record attendance and sickness absence. Occupational health services have an important role to play in advising on the management of sickness absence and should be involved with management in the planning, implementation and assessment of any initiatives.

Effort is needed to achieve real improvements in the state of employees' health. Despite the obvious commercial benefits, a Health Education Authority (HEA) study of health promotion in 1,344 workplaces in England[2] found that only 40% of workplaces undertook some health promotion activity. Larger workplaces were more likely to have some form of health promotion and to cover a wider range of issues, but 60% of firms with less than 24 employees had no health promotion programmes and, even in companies with over 500 employees, only 25% had five or more health promotion programmes in operation.

Companies are now obliged to be able to assess risks to the health and safety of their workforce[3], and personnel managers need to take into account the effects that mental or physical ill-health can have on employees' performance at work. Efficiency on health and safety issues correlates with overall business efficiency: companies that control health and safety risks and reduce absenteeism through ill-health may also improve productivity and reduce staff turnover.

References

1. Confederation of British Industry, BUPA. *Working for your health: practical steps to improve the health of your business.* London: Confederation of British Industry, 1993.
2. Health Education Authority. *Health Promotion in the Workplace: a summary.* London: Health Education Authority, 1993.
3. Health and Safety Commission. *Management of Health and Safety at Work: management of Health and Safety at Work Regulations 1992: approved code of practice.* London: HMSO, 1992.

(e)   Urban health

Concern about the health of people who live in towns and cities is not a new phenomenon. In the middle of the last century, the Health of Towns Association was set up in response to perceived threats to the public health posed by industrialisation and rapid urbanisation, and helped to change the poor living conditions of many people who lived in towns and cities. More recently, the possible consequences of a relative increase in urban populations in western and developing countries have been widely discussed.

Urbanisation not only leads to an increased population density within a given geographical area, but influences means of governance and culture and alters the social and physical infrastructure[1]. However, even within towns and cities there are striking contrasts between the local environments, neighbourhoods, localities and communities. The effects on health and health service delivery are just as complex[2].

International research into the health of people in cities, especially the urban poor, has identified three groups of factors which may contribute to poor health[3]. The first group include the direct effects of low income or limited education. Next are man-made conditions, such as overcrowding; poor housing and sanitation; and industrialisation, pollution and increased exposure to occupational diseases. Finally, there are the social and psychological consequences of a rapid turnover of people, loss of social supports and increasing social isolation.

The World Health Organization's (WHO's) 'Healthy Cities Project'[4] was launched in 1986, with collaboration between cities to develop local action plans for health promotion, using community participation together with a partnership between the public, private and voluntary sectors to focus on urban health. The strategy for health recognises the importance of urban health and has identified 'healthy cities' as one of its healthy settings[5]. DH also supports the UK 'Health for All Network' which helps to link together local projects to improve health.

Urban health is not just relevant to England or the UK but has global implications for public health and health services delivery. At the beginning of the 19th century, the world's urban population was less than 50 million people;

by 1990 it exceeded 1.6 billion and the United Nations predicts a figure of 3.1 billion by the year 2000. Increased attention must be paid to the impact of an urban environment and lifestyle on health, and the ways to enhance any beneficial, and to counteract any harmful, effects.

References

1. Duhl L. *Healthy Cities: myth or reality?* In: Ashton J, ed. *Healthy Cities.* Buckingham: Open University Press, 1992.
2. Benzeval M, Judge K, Soboman M. *The Health Status of Londoners: a comparative perspective.* London: King's Fund Institute, 1992.
3. Harpham T, Lusty T, Vaughan P, eds. *In the Shadow of the City: community health and the urban poor.* Oxford: Oxford University Press, 1988.
4. Davies JK, Kelly MP, eds. *Healthy cities: research and practice.* London: Routledge, 1993.
5. Department of Health. *The Health of the Nation: a strategy for health in England.* London: HMSO, 1992 (Cm. 1986).

(f)   Variations in health

Significant variations in health may be observed in relation to geographical area, ethnicity, social class, occupation and gender. Such variations, which occur within England and internationally, are a cause for concern if there is no known reason for their existence, and a challenge because they indicate that there is scope for improvement. Even when a reason for their existence can be identified, interventions to bring about improvements may be difficult to achieve.

These problems can be illustrated if accidents are used as an example. Of 9,644 accidental deaths in England during 1992, about 59% were in men and only 41% among women - a sex ratio of 1.4:1. People in social class V are five times more likely to die as the result of an accident than those in social class I, and death rates from accidents appear to be higher among unemployed men than among those who have a job. Mortality rates from motor vehicle traffic accidents are higher in rural than in urban areas. One study also found significantly more road accidents involving pedestrians among Asian children than in the white population[1], although the authors concluded that age and the type of road on which accidents occurred had a greater effect than ethnic origin.

Thus variations in health may be complex and inter-related, and causal factors may only be identified by a careful assessment of all available evidence. Even when causes can be identified, the impact of interventions intended to reduce these variations may be unpredictable. The need for further scientifically based and well evaluated research has been recognised by the establishment of a subgroup of the Chief Medical Officer's Health of the Nation Working Group to examine specific aspects of variations in health that relate to targets in the strategy for health[2].

References

1. Lawson SD. *Accidents to young pedestrians: distribution, circumstances, consequences and scope for countermeasures.* Basingstoke (Hampshire): AA Foundation for Road Safety Research and Birmingham City Council, 1990.
2. Department of Health. *The Health of the Nation: a strategy for health in England.* London: HMSO, 1992 (Cm. 1986).

(g) Health of people in later life

As was appropriate for the 'European Year of Older People and Solidarity between Generations', 1993 saw several developments relevant to the health care requirements of older people. DH organised an inter-disciplinary workshop on osteoarthritis in February, which reviewed current knowledge on connective tissue ageing and osteoarthritis and its relevance to the health of older people in the UK and suggested research priorities to contribute to the development of strategies for the prevention and treatment of osteoarthritis in old age. As a result, DH will be commissioning further research into primary care interventions in osteoarthritis. DH also considered the implications for health and social policies of projected demographic changes to the elderly population, described in last year's Report[1]. The proceedings of a series of workshops held to assess these changes during 1993 should be published in 1994.

DH contributed to a Royal College of Physicians of London Working Party on the interface between geriatric and general medicine. The Working Party concentrated on the interface between geriatric and general internal medicine in relation to acute emergency care, specialist care, training and research, and the commissioning and provision of health care services for older people[2].

A workshop on stroke rehabilitation, organised in partnership with the Nuffield Hospital Provincial Trust, was held in October. The aims of the workshop were to define and advise on the key issues and components in stroke rehabilitation, and to identify future research strategies and policies for care. Evidence presented at the workshop indicated that co-ordinated management of stroke by a multidisciplinary team of professionals was cost-effective and could help to reduce mortality and expedite recovery from stroke.

The Royal College of Psychiatrists held two conferences in November that were funded by DH. The first, organised in association with the British Geriatrics Society, discussed joint approaches to the assessment, long-stay care, and management of chronic disease and elder abuse. The second, organised in association with the Alzheimer's Disease Society, the Royal College of General Practitioners and Age Concern, discussed the organisation and co-ordination of services needed for older people with dementia.

As part of the implementation of *Caring for People*[3], DH organised a series of workshops to prepare ground rules to enable purchasers and providers to organise effective discharge from hospital. A manual on hospital discharge practice will be published in Spring 1994.

At the end of November, the All-Party Group on Ageing held a seminar at the House of Lords on Health for Older People. The meeting, chaired by Lord Stallard, was addressed by Baroness Cumberlege, Parliamentary Under Secretary of State for Health in the House of Lords, and included presentations from Age Concern, dietitians and the leisure industry, and looked at relevant aspects of health care and epidemiology.

References

1. Department of Health. *On the State of the Public Health: the annual report of the Chief Medical Officer of the Department of Health for the Year 1992.* London: HMSO, 1993: 135-8.
2. Royal College of Physicians of London. *Equity of Care: the interface between geriatric medicine and internal medicine.* London: Royal College of Physicians (in press).
3. Department of Health. *Caring for People: community care in the next decade and beyond.* London: HMSO, 1989.

(h)   Health of black and ethnic minorities

The Report for 1991[1] drew attention to some of the differences in health and disease patterns seen in people from black and ethnic minority communities and highlighted the difficulties in access to health services experienced by some ethnic groups.

The Ethnic Health Unit

During 1993, Baroness Cumberlege, Parliamentary Under Secretary of State for Health in the House of Lords, established a Task Force to produce a report on action needed to improve NHS services for black and ethnic communities[2]. As a result, an Ethnic Health Unit was established within the NHS Management Executive. This small multidisciplinary team is supported by a group of experts and representatives from ethnic community organisations. An extra £500,000 will be available for health authorities to support initiatives by local organisations, to supplement £800,000 in grants that the Department already gives to community organisations[3].

Surveys and research

Last year's Report[4] described research into accident prevention, which was completed and published[5]. Work started on the Fourth National Survey of Ethnic Minorities, a decennial survey of the economic and social conditions of Britain's larger ethnic groups by the Policy Studies Institute, which for the first time includes a section on health. Preparatory work for a survey of infant feeding among the Asian population was also undertaken.

Policy development

Much of the work described elsewhere in this Report will affect the health of people in ethnic minority groups. The importance of ethnicity was highlighted in general policy development: the publication of *User Sensitive Purchasing*[6] outlines specific aspects of the purchasing process that all parts of the NHS need to consider when purchasing for ethnic communities. *Building on Strengths*[7] describes the Asian voluntary sector in England. An understanding of the voluntary sector among ethnic communities is important for the development of services sensitive to local needs, and *Health for all our children*[8] and *Access to Health Care*[9] both set standards for health care services for patients from black and ethnic minority groups.

Achievement of the overall population targets set in the strategy for health[10] will require the active involvement of members of black and ethnic minority groups, and the report *Ethnicity and Health*[11] highlights the importance of Health of the Nation key areas for different ethnic groups.

The report of the Standing Medical Advisory Committee (SMAC) Working Party on sickle cell, thalassaemia and other haemoglobinopathies was endorsed by SMAC and presented to the Secretary of State for Health. Publication is likely early in 1994.

Ethnic monitoring

Work continued towards the implementation of ethnic monitoring as part of the NHS inpatient data set, including work on the development of practical guidance on data collection, as well as consultation exercises.

Equal opportunities for NHS staff

In December, the Secretary of State for Health launched a programme of action to promote equal opportunities in the NHS for staff from ethnic minorities based on advice received by a Working Group that she chaired. The programme sets out goals, for the achievement of which the Chairmen or Chairwomen and Chief Executives of Health Authorities and Trusts within the NHS will be held accountable.

References

1. Department of Health. *On the State of the Public Health: the annual report of the Chief Medical Officer of the Department of Health for the year 1991.* London: HMSO, 1992; 8-9, 54-77.
2. Department of Health. *Baroness Cumberlege announces initiative to improve health and services for black and ethnic people.* London: Department of Health, 1993 (Press Release: H93/912).
3. Department of Health. *NHS Ethnic Unit, Leeds.* Heywood (Lancashire): Department of Health, 1993 (Executive Letter: EL(93)89).
4. Department of Health. *On the State of the Public Health: the annual report of the Chief Medical Officer for the Department of Health for the year 1992.* London: HMSO, 1993: 18-19; 138-49.
5. Parmar A. *Safety and minority ethnic communities: a preliminary report on the home safety information needs of the Asian, Chinese and Vietnamese communities living in the UK in the 1990s.* Birmingham: Royal Society for the Prevention of Accidents, 1993.
6. Mohammed S. *User sensitive purchasing.* London: King's Fund Centre, 1993.
7. Webb-Johnson A. *Building on Strengths: inquiry into the health activity in the Asian voluntary sector.* London: Confederation of Indian Organisations, 1993.
8. Slater M. *Health for all our children: achieving appropriate health care for black and ethnic minority children.* London: Action for Sick Children, 1993.
9. Hopkins A, Bahl V. *Access to health care for people from black and ethnic minorities.* London: Royal College of Physicians, 1993.
10. Department of Health. *The Health of the Nation: a strategy for health in England.* London: Department of Health, 1992 (Cm. 1986).
11. Balarajan R, Soni Raleigh V. *Ethnicity and Health: a guide for the NHS.* London: Department of Health, 1993.

(i) Health of men

Last year's Report[1] described some of the differences in health and lifestyle between men and women, although it stressed that many of the major causes of death and illness were similar in men and women alike, on review of available mortality and morbidity data. Data now available for 1991-92 from the 4th Morbidity Survey in General Practice[2] (MSGP-4) show little change in the general pattern of consultations since the 3rd survey in 1981-82[3], referred to in last year's Report[1], and any changes (for example a slight increase in consultations for injuries and diseases of the skin and subcutaneous tissues among young adults) need to be treated with caution because of shifts in attendance patterns between primary and secondary care.

Accidents

Among people aged 15-24 years, four times as many men die from accidents as women. Road traffic accidents account for some 70% of these accidental deaths which are often associated with alcohol and driver inexperience. Nevertheless, encouraging progress has been made towards the targets set out in the strategy for health[4]: a 5.2% reduction towards the overall target of a 25% reduction in deaths among this age-group before the year 2005 was seen for 1992 data. The Department of Transport's Drink Driving programme has contributed to this reduction and further progress should be made as a result of their safety initiative for new drivers.

Mental illness

Young men who commit suicide appear to be less likely to consult their general practitioner in the preceding month than women and other age-groups[5]. Strategies to reduce access to means of committing suicide and ways to encourage young men to seek help when depressed are being reviewed.

Health and work

Men make up just over 51% of the employed workforce of 21 million people and the workplace is a useful setting to encourage health promotion. Recommendations of the Workplace Task Force[6], which was set up to take forward work on healthy workplaces as part of the strategy for health initiative[4], included the need for better evaluation of workplace health promotional activity, and more effective communication about good practice and the availability of appropriate health promotion material. The Task Force also advised the establishment of local alliance groups comprising representatives from health promotion, occupational health, and health and safety organisations as well as chambers of commerce to provide information, advice and support for employers who wanted to increase their health promotion activities. Three pilot local alliance groups were established during 1993 in Manchester, Sheffield, and Winchester and their activities will be evaluated during 1994.

The way ahead

Some local initiatives have specifically targeted the health needs of men. These include the Everyman centre in South London, a charity which aims to stop physical and social violence through individual and group counselling and support services (including a helpline), and to enable men to examine and re-evaluate their attitudes to masculinity, sexuality, relationships and violent behaviour; an academic research programme helps to measure the effectiveness of the project on violent behaviour. The East Midlands Men's Health Network, a forum open to men and women who care for men in a range of settings, provides relevant books, leaflets, training packs and videos available on loan. A review of sexual health initiatives for heterosexual men for the HEA looked at three geographical areas and used known men's health networks to try to identify such initiatives across the country: examples identified included an information project for young people in Waltham Forest, which covers not only health but leisure, careers and training, and rights and benefits. Other projects include a testicular cancer support group in Southampton and cardiac clubs for men (and women) who have had heart attacks.

In the long run such local initiatives to improve men's health and the services available to them should lead to healthier lifestyles, improved health and greater life expectancy.

References

1. Department of Health. *On the State of the Public Health: the annual report of the Chief Medical Officer of the Department of Health for the year 1992.* London: HMSO, 1993; 79-106.
2. Office of Population Censuses and Surveys. *Morbidity Statistics from General Practice 1991-92 (MSGP-4).* London: HMSO (in press).
3. Office of Population Censuses and Surveys. *Morbidity Statistics from General Practice 1981-82 (MSGP-3).* London: HMSO, 1986 (OPCS Monitor MB5 no. 1).
4. Department of Health. *The Health of the Nation: a strategy for health in England.* London: HMSO, 1992 (Cm. 1986).
5. Vassilas CA, Morgan HG. General practitioners' contact with victims of suicide. *BMJ* 1993; **307:** 300-1.
6. Department of Health. *Health of the Nation: Workplace Task Force report.* London: Department of Health, 1993. Chair: Mr Terry Hogg.

CHAPTER 3

THE STRATEGY FOR HEALTH

(a)   One year on

The White Paper *The Health of the Nation: a strategy for health in England*[1] was published in July 1992. Details of the targets and the strategy were given in last year's Report[2]. The main priority during the strategy's first year of operation has been to ensure the commitment and support of all sections of the community, including other Government Departments, the National Health Service (NHS) and other national and local organisations. Progress was summarised in the report *One Year On*[3], published in November.

The three Working Groups set up to help develop the strategy for health, chaired by Baroness Cumberlege, Parliamentary Under Secretary of State for Health in the House of Lords, the Chief Medical Officer, and the NHS Chief Executive, continue to assist in its implementation. Work in the specific areas of nutrition, smoking, accidents, the workplace, physical activity and mental illness is being developed by individual Task Forces.

As part of a programme of support for all those who help to deliver health care within the NHS, handbooks were produced on each of the five key areas (coronary heart disease [CHD] and stroke[4], cancers[5], mental illness[6], HIV/AIDS and sexual health[7] and accidents[8]), on ethnic health issues[9] and on the role of nurses, midwives and health visitors[10]. For those working both within and outside the health service, the setting up of alliances for health was described in *Working Together for Better Health*[11], prepared under the guidance of the Wider Health Working Group. A quarterly newsletter, *Target*, is circulated widely within and outside the NHS to disseminate activities and ideas associated with the Health of the Nation initiative. A special update is included in each monthly edition of *NHS Management Executive News*.

The value of local initiatives was emphasised in a series of 14 regional conferences, held early in 1993. To mark the first anniversary of the initiative, a special youth conference with the theme 'Listening to the Next Generation' was held in London and was addressed by the Secretary of State for Health.

The role of voluntary organisations in promoting health has not been overlooked. Extra funding has been made available to 13 agencies under Section 64 arrangements of the Health Services and Public Health Act 1968[12]: £250,000 were allocated in 1992/93, and £260,000 have been made available for 1993/94.

During 1993, work continued to monitor progress towards the primary targets of the strategy[1], as set out in the *Specification of National Indicators*[13], and to identify and monitor supplementary indicators of progress. To aid monitoring at a local level, four releases of the Public Health Common Data Set were made during 1993, including an analysis of mortality trends since 1984[14,15,16,17]. Epidemiological overviews on CHD and stroke will be published early in 1994. The first Health Survey Report[18] was published in July 1993, and is described on page 113. At its launch, the Chief Medical Officer issued a challenge to the nation comprising 20 simple steps that can be taken by anyone to improve their own health. Work started towards the end of the year to re-launch the challenge and to secure a wider distribution nationwide.

References

1. Department of Health. *The Health of the Nation: a strategy for health in England.* London: HMSO, 1992 (Cm. 1986).
2. Department of Health. *On the State of the Public Health: the annual report of the Chief Medical Officer of the Department of Health for the year 1992.* London: HMSO, 1993: 10-11, 66-78.
3. Department of Health. *Health of the Nation: one year on - a report on the progress of the Health of the Nation.* London: Department of Health, 1993.
4. Department of Health. *The Health of the Nation Key Area Handbook: coronary heart disease and stroke.* London: Department of Health, 1993.
5. Department of Health. *Health of the Nation Key Area Handbook: cancers.* London: Department of Health, 1993.
6. Department of Health. *Health of the Nation Key Area Handbook: mental illness.* London: Department of Health, 1993.
7. Department of Health. *Health of the Nation Key Area Handbook: HIV/AIDS and sexual health.* London: Department of Health, 1993.
8. Department of Health. *Health of the Nation Key Area Handbook: accidents.* London: Department of Health, 1993.
9. Department of Health. *Ethnicity and Health: a guide for the NHS.* Heywood (Lancashire): Department of Health, 1993.
10. Department of Health. *Targeting Practice: the contribution of nurses, midwives and health visitors.* London: Department of Health, 1993.
11. Department of Health. *Working Together for Better Health.* London: Department of Health, 1993.
12. *Health Services and Public Health Act 1968.* London: HMSO, 1968.
13. Department of Health. *Specification of National Indicators.* London: Department of Health, 1992.
14. Department of Health. *Public health common data set 1993: incorporating indicators from the Health of the Nation (based on data for years up to 1992): data definitions and user guide for computer files.* Guildford: Institute of Public Health, 1993. (Mortality data; vol 1.)
15. Department of Health. *Public health common data set 1993: incorporating indicators from the Health of the Nation (based on data for years up to 1992): data definitions and user guide for computer files.* Guildford: Institute of Public Health, 1993. (Demography, fertility, morbidity and determinants of health; vol 2.)
16. Department of Health. *Public health common data set 1993: data definitions and user guide for computer files.* Guildford: Institute of Public Health, 1993. (1991 Census supplement; vol 3.)
17. Department of Health. *Public health common data set 1993: incorporating indicators from the Health of the Nation (based on data for years up to 1992): data definitions and user guide for computer files.* Guildford: Institute of Public Health, 1993. (Mortality trend data (based on Census rebased population estimates); vol 4.)
18. Office of Population Censuses and Surveys. *Health Survey for England 1991.* London: HMSO, 1993.

(b)   Key areas and targets

(i)   *Coronary heart disease and stroke*

Action to achieve the CHD/stroke targets includes the general 'Look After Your Heart' (LAYH) programme as well as specific initiatives for the individual major risk factors (hypertension, raised cholesterol [see page 69], smoking [see page 65] and lack of physical activity. Risk factors for CHD were analysed in the 1991 Health Survey for England[1], published in 1993, and will be followed up over the next three years: only 12% of men and 11% of women were free from all four of the major risk factors of hypertension, hypercholesterolaemia, cigarette smoking and low levels of physical activity.

The book *Better Living, Better Life*[2] was commissioned by the Chief Medical Officer's Tripartite Group on Effective Health Promotion in Primary Care (which includes representatives of the General Medical Services Committee of the British Medical Association, the Royal College of General Practitioners, and the Department of Health [DH]). It sets out guidance on effective interventions to reduce CHD and stroke and was distributed to all general practices in England. The key area handbook for CHD and stroke[3] also gives practical advice and examples of good practice aimed at managers and professionals alike, and includes a statement of Government policy on cholesterol testing subsequent to the Standing Medical Advisory Committee's report on the cost-effectiveness of opportunistic cholesterol screening in general practice. In outline, cholesterol testing should be offered to individuals as part of an overall CHD prevention programme, including appropriate interventions, based on case-finding of those at increased risk of CHD. An Effective Health Care Bulletin[4] on cholesterol screening and treatment was published in June.

CHD and stroke were the focus of new arrangements for health promotion within the general practitioner (GP) contract, implemented from 1 July. Practices elect whether to take part and can choose from three levels of involvement: band 1 programmes seek to reduce smoking; band 2 to minimise morbidity and mortality of patients at high risk from hypertension or with pre-existing CHD or stroke; and practices in band 3 offer a full range of primary prevention for CHD and stroke according to the needs of their practice population, including advice on diet, physical activity and alcohol intake. More than 90% of GPs are in band 3.

Physical Activity

Following a commitment in the White Paper[5] to develop detailed strategies for physical activity in the light of the findings of the Allied Dunbar National Fitness Survey[6], a Health of the Nation Task force was announced in July to advise on the setting of specific targets for physical activity which might form the basis of such strategies.

Alcohol

The 1992 General Household Survey[7] (GHS) showed that 26% of men drink more than the recommended sensible level of 21 units per week, and 12% of women drink more than 14 units; these findings are not significantly different from those in 1990[8]. Over one-third of young men aged 18-24 years drink more than 21 units per week. A survey of attitudes to, and knowledge of, sensible drinking limits[9] indicates increased public awareness of these guidelines: 46% of men and 48% of women who drank alcohol had a reasonable idea of the limits, and 26% of all men and 36% of all women had exact knowledge.

The LAYH strategy will be revised to take account of the strategy for health's CHD and stroke targets for people aged 65-74 years[5]. In 1993, LAYH contributed to the Family Smoking Campaign, a major pilot project in the north of England to help parents to stop smoking cigarettes and to discourage their children from starting to smoke.

(ii)   Cancers

The Health of the Nation White Paper[5] focused on breast cancer, cervical cancer, skin cancer and lung cancer - four major cancers which account for about 35% of all cancer deaths.

Breast cancer

A reduction in the death rate for female breast cancer in the population invited for screening by at least 25% from 1990 figures will require effective implementation of the national screening programme as early detection offers the best prognosis. In 1991/92, 1.4 million women were invited for breast cancer screening, of whom 1.02 million accepted their invitations and among whom 6,605 cancers were detected[10,11]. By the end of 1993, 93% of all eligible women should have been invited for breast cancer screening. However, acceptance rates vary from area to area - from 80% in some suburban and rural areas to as little as 50% in parts of inner cities. The challenges now are to increase the number of women being screened; to evaluate the screening programme; and to pursue research into breast cancer screening and treatment.

Cervical cancer

Early changes in the cervix which may lead to cancer can generally be detected by examination of cells scraped easily from its surface. In 1991/92, 1.19 million women were invited for screening in the national cervical screening programme; over 80% of these women had been screened in the previous 5.5 years. However, public confidence in the screening could have been weakened by reports in the later part of the year that some smears had not been taken by the recommended method in a small number of general practices.

It is vital that public confidence is maintained. New guidelines[12], issued in August, updated earlier guidance on the running of the programme, and primary health care teams were reminded[13] of the need to ensure training and professional competence when tasks are delegated. The National Co-ordinating Network, described in the key area handbook on cancers[14], is developing quality standards for the programme which should be published during 1994 and management of the national programme is under review.

Skin cancer

The key area handbook on cancers[14] contains guidance for the National Health Service (NHS) on how to establish local skin cancer prevention initiatives during the year, and identifies three main objectives:

- to increase the number of people who are aware of their own skin cancer risk factors;

- to persuade people at high risk to avoid excessive exposure to the sun and artificial sources of ultraviolet (UV) radiation for themselves and for their children, through changes in behaviour and use of sun protection measures; *and*

- to alter people's attitudes to a tanned appearance.

All GPs were sent a letter[15] in July to draw their attention to the skin cancer target and to new public information on avoiding excessive UV radiation. A survey by the Office of Population Censuses and Surveys (OPCS) showed that large numbers of the public lack knowledge about skin cancer and sun avoidance measures. Weekly public reports of ground level UV radiation are now available from the National Radiological Protection Board.

Lung cancer

Smoking remains the major risk factor for lung cancer. The prevalence of cigarette smoking among adults continues to fall, from nearly 30% in 1990 to about 28% in 1992 (see Table 3.1); the target is a prevalence of not more than 20% in the year 2000. By June 1993, total consumption of cigarettes had fallen by around 10% compared with the 1990 baseline; the target is a 40% reduction by the year 2000. The proportion of women smokers who stop smoking during pregnancy is increasing towards the target of 1 in 3.

Whilst smoking prevalence among adults continues to fall, smoking among children aged 11-15 years is virtually unchanged at 10% (see Table 3.2). Although the social acceptability of smoking is falling, a greater reduction in adult smoking may be required before teenagers' attitudes are significantly affected. There is still a long way to go to reach the target of below 6% smoking prevalence in this age-group by the end of 1994. The 1992 figures do not reflect price increases in the two 1993 Budgets or full implementation of new laws on illegal sales of tobacco to children, but extra effort is clearly needed. Action will continue to encourage everyone concerned - parents, teachers, youth workers, trading standards officers and health professionals - to redouble their efforts to reduce smoking among children.

Although young people will continue to be addressed through health education programmes, it is increasingly recognised that family example is an important factor in teenage smoking and health education campaigns aimed at adults are being broadened to help parents give up smoking to reduce risks to their children.

Further evidence of the harmful effects of passive smoking was given in a report by the United States (US) Environmental Protection Agency[16], which highlighted the harmful effects of tobacco smoke on children. Continued progress has been made in the implementation of non-smoking policies in public places but there is still room for improvement. The NHS smoke-free policy was in place by the middle of the year.

Table 3.1: *Prevalence of cigarette smoking in adults (aged 16 years and over) in England, 1974-92*

Year	Men %	Women %
1974	51	40
1978	44	36
1982	37	32
1984	35	32
1986	34	31
1988	32	30
1990	31	28
1992	29	27
2000 target	*20*	*20*

Source: OPCS (GHS)

Table 3.2: *Prevalence of regular* cigarette smoking in children (aged 11-15 years) in England, 1982-1993*

Year	Boys %	Girls %	Total %
1982	11	11	11
1984	13	13	13
1986	7	12	10
1988	7	9	8
1990	9	11	10
1992	9	10	10
1993†	8	11	10
1994 target			*<6*

* Regular smoking defined as usually smoking at least one cigarette per week.
† Provisional data.

Source: OPCS

(iii) Mental illness

Steady progress has been made towards the objectives set out for mental illness in the Health of the Nation White Paper[5]. A Departmental steering committee was set up in 1992 to drive forward and to co-ordinate work; the key area handbook[17], published in January, sets out a comprehensive agenda to help the NHS and its partners in alliances for mental health to achieve the objectives. Work has continued on technical aspects of measuring the main targets. The Brief Standardised Assessment Procedure to measure the health and social functioning of mentally ill people is being assessed by the Research Unit of the Royal College of Psychiatrists, and should be available for wider use in clinical practice by 1996. Guidelines to support the clinical audit of suicide and other unexpected deaths have been commissioned. The national suicide rate for the triennium to December 1992 showed a small increase on the figures for 1989-91, underlining the need for accurate assessment and effective preventive measures.

A survey of public attitudes to people with mental illness showed broad support for the principles of community care, but highlighted the need to increase public awareness and understanding of mental illness to reduce its stigma. Three booklets to help to explain mental illness - *What does it mean?*[18], *A guide to mental health in the workplace*[19] and *Sometimes I think I can't go on anymore*[20] - were published and a series of exhibitions about mental health in the workplace were mounted.

Policy on the care of people with severe and enduring mental illness was comprehensively reviewed, and a study of the factors that influence implementation of the Care Programme Approach was published[21], as was a review of legal aspects of the care of patients outside hospital[22]. The Secretary of State for Health announced a ten-point plan to reinforce community care for mentally ill people, which included the introduction of a new power of supervised discharge, development of a training programme for key workers, reviews of guidelines for the discharge of patients from psychiatric hospitals and for the treatment of schizophrenia, and the setting up of supervision registers for some patients who are being cared for in community settings. Taken together, these developments should improve the health and social functioning of many mentally ill people, and enable more effective supervision of those for whom the risk of relapse carries a real possibility of serious self-neglect or violent or suicidal behaviour.

(iv)   HIV/AIDS and sexual health

The *Health of the Nation* White Paper[5] includes objectives to reduce the incidence of HIV infection and other sexually transmitted diseases (STDs) and to reduce unwanted pregnancies. Reports of new cases of gonorrhoea in England fell by 7.4% in 1991 and by a further 24% in 1992[23], which indicates that behavioural change may have occurred among groups most at risk from all STDs including HIV infection. The 1992 figure for new cases is below the target set for 1995. The percentage of notified drug misusers who inject drugs also fell from 60% in 1991 to 56% in 1992. Ways to monitor progress towards targets for reduced equipment sharing by injecting drug users are being developed with health authorities and other agencies.

In 1991, the conception rate among girls aged under 16 years fell for the first time in 10 years from 10.1 to 9.3 per 1,000. Teenage abortion rates have also fallen from 19.6 per 1,000 in 1988 to 16.9 in 1992. Abortion rates for all ages fell by 3.8% in 1991 - the first fall since 1983 - and by another 4.2% in 1992.

DH is working closely with the NHS and others to sustain progress towards targets in this key area. The HIV/AIDS and sexual health handbook[24], published in 1993, provides advice and practical examples to assist the development of realistic local sexual health and drug misuse prevention strategies. In 1993/94, DH provided over £31 million for HIV prevention and sexual health promotion and over £24 million to combat drug misuse, including £2.6 million to expand needle exchange schemes. Grants have also been made to a wide range of organisations concerned with HIV prevention and drug misuse services.

NHS health authorities are now required to provide a full range of family planning services[25], with particular attention to emergency contraception and services for young people. DH continues to work with voluntary bodies such as the Family Planning Association, the Brook Advisory Centres and the Sex Education Forum, and has collaborated with the English National Board on a sexual health education conference held in March to encourage debate among nursing professionals. The Royal College of Obstetricians and Gynaecologists established a Faculty of Family Planning and the College's Teenage Pregnancy Steering Group took forward initiatives to support the strategy for health's targets.

Continued work and support is necessary if early progress towards targets is to be maintained and improved. In particular, the momentum of local and national HIV/STD prevention must be maintained to emphasise the need for safer sex, and family planning information and services must be further improved to reduce the numbers of unwanted conceptions to the targets set out in the White Paper[5].

(v)   Accidents

Accidental injury is an important cause of death, disability and ill health, and encouraging progress has already been made towards the targets to reduce accident mortality set out in the *Health of the Nation* White Paper[5]. In 1992, death rates from accidents fell by 6.8% among children, by 16.2% among young people aged 15-24 years and by 6.8% among people aged 65 years and older. Incorporation of these figures into the three-year moving averages for 1990-92 shows progress of 9.0% towards the 33% reduction sought for children, of 4.8% towards the 25% reduction sought for young adults, and of 5.0% towards the 33% reduction sought for people aged 65 years and older.

However, injuries caused by accidents far exceed deaths, and the full benefit of the prevention strategy will only be known when trends in morbidity and long-term disability can be monitored. The national accident prevention Task Force has therefore made the improvement of the range and compatibility of information collected about accidental injuries one of its main priorities. This Task Force was established in 1992 and includes representatives of 11

Government Departments, three voluntary organisations, the media, emergency services, the NHS, local authorities and industry. Sub-groups, to which external specialists have been co-opted, were established in 1993 to report on information and research needs and the role in accident prevention of medical and nursing staff who work in accident and emergency departments.

A study by the Department's Public Health Information Strategy team indicates that better information on the causes, severity and long-term consequences of accidental injuries might be obtained by the further development and linkage of existing data sources (unpublished). There will be wide consultation about the implementation of these recommendations. Another preliminary study indicates that more consistency is needed when defining research objectives and findings, and that evaluation of current accident prevention practice should command priority in future research programmes.

Plans for additional work with other agencies include increased integration of accident prevention with other relevant aspects of health promotion, such as misuse of drugs and alcohol; collaboration on policy development elsewhere in the NHS, such as the use of health checks for older people to identify risk factors for accidental injury; and support of accident prevention initiatives by the Institution of Environmental Health Officers.

References

1. Office of Population Censuses and Surveys. *Health Survey for England 1991*. London: HMSO, 1993.
2. Department of Health, British Medical Association, Royal College of General Practitioners: *Better Living, Better Life*. Henley-on-Thames: Knowledge House Ltd, 1993.
3. Department of Health. *The Health of the Nation Key Area Handbook: coronary heart disease and stroke*. London: Department of Health, 1993.
4. Freemantle N, Long A, Mason J, Sheldon T, Song F, Wison C. Cholesterol: screening and treatment. *Effective Health Care* 1993; **6**: 1-16.
5. Department of Health. *The Health of the Nation: a strategy for health in England*. London: HMSO, 1992 (Cm. 1986).
6. Allied Dunbar National Fitness Survey. *A report on activity patterns and fitness levels commissioned by the Sports Council and the Health Education Authority: main findings*. London: Sports Council, 1992.
7. Office of Population Censuses and Surveys. *General Household Survey 1992*. London: HMSO (in press).
8. Office of Population Censuses and Surveys. *General Household Survey 1990*. London: HMSO, 1992 (GHS no. 22).
9. Office of Population Censuses and Surveys. *Omnibus Survey of Drinking in Great Britain: February and March 1993*. OPCS: HMSO (in press).
10. Department of Health. *Breast Cancer Screening 1991/92: summary information from form KC62*: England. London: Department of Health, 1993.
11. Trent Regional Health Authority. *National Health Service Breast Screening Programme: review 1993*. Sheffield: Trent RHA, 1993.
12. Department of Health. *National cervical screening programme*. Heywood (Lancashire): Department of Health, 1993 (Health Service Guidelines: HSG(93)41).
13. Department of Health. *Professional Responsibility, Accountability and Delegation of Tasks*. Heywood (Lancashire): Department of Health, 1993 (Professional Letter: PL/CMO(93)14; PL(CNO(93)6).
14. Department of Health. *The Health of the Nation Key Area Handbook: cancers*. London: Department of Health 1993; 127-8, 138-40, 143.
15. Department of Health. *Ultraviolet radiation and skin cancer*. Heywood (Lancashire): Department of Health, 1993 (Professional Letter: PL/CMO(93)6).
16. United States Environmental Protection Agency. *Respiratory health effects of passive smoking: lung cancer and other disorders*. Ohio, USA: US Environmental Protection Agency, 1992 (EPA/600/6-90/006F).
17. Department of Health. *The Health of the Nation Key Area Handbook: mental illness*. London: Department of Health, 1993.
18. Department of Health. *The Health of the Nation: mental illness. What does it mean?* Heywood (Lancashire): Department of Health, 1993.
19. Department of Health. *The Health of the Nation: mental illness: a guide to mental health in the workplace*.

London: Department of Health, 1993.

20. Department of Health. *The Health of the Nation: mental illness. Sometimes I think I can't go on anymore.* Heywood (Lancashire): Department of Health, 1993.

21. North C, Ritchie J, Ward K. *Factors Influencing the Implementation of the Care Programme Approach: a research study carried out for the Department of Health by Social and Community Planning Research.* London: HMSO, 1993.

22. Department of Health. *Legal powers on the care of mentally ill people in the Community: report of the internal review.* London: Department of Health, 1993. Chairs: Miss Dora Pease, Dr John Reed.

23. Department of Health. *On the State of the Public Health: the annual report of the Chief Medical Officer for the year 1992.* London: HMSO, 1993; 160-4.

24. Department of Health. *The Health of the Nation Key Area Handbook: HIV/AIDS and sexual health.* London: Department of Health, 1993.

25. NHS Management Executive. *Priorities and Planning Guidance 1994/95.* Heywood (Lancashire): Department of Health, 1993 (Executive Letter: EL(93)54).

(c) Nutrition

The *Health of the Nation* White Paper[1] contained dietary and nutritional targets within the key area of CHD and stroke: a reduced intake of fat and saturated fatty acids, and a reduction in adult obesity. Lower salt intake is also seen as a necessary contribution to achieving the national target to reduce blood pressure. In December 1992, a Nutrition Task Force chaired by Professor Dame Barbara Clayton was set up to prepare an action programme to help to achieve these nutrition targets.

In 1993, this Task Force prepared outline proposals and priorities for action which were approved by Ministers in DH and the Ministry of Agriculture, Fisheries and Food (MAFF), and were issued for public consultation in June[2]. Over 180 responses were received. In October, the Task Force adopted a final programme of action modified in the light of the consultation, which was agreed by DH and MAFF Ministers in December 1993 and will be published in Spring 1994. The programme contains proposals for: appropriate criteria for nutrition education materials; a review of advertising codes of practice; nutrition in school curricula and the setting up of a General Certificate of Secondary Education (GCSE) examination in food and nutrition; nutritional guidelines for caterers in schools, hospitals, workplaces, and the fast-food sector; nutritional training for caterers; a food industry review of the fat content of manufactured products; reduction of fat in animal and poultry carcasses; promotion of healthy foods; a nutrition handbook for NHS managers; a core nutrition curriculum document for education of health professionals; nutrition guidance for primary health care teams; the education of dietitians and nutritionists; and research into effective interventions. Special attention will be paid to the problems of people on low incomes, those in ethnic minority groups and older people.

In the White Paper[1], the Government promised "to continue and enhance research into the links between diet and health, and into influences on consumer choice". DH, in association with the Medical Research Council (MRC), has convened a Nutrition Programme Committee to co-ordinate research in human nutrition to support these responsibilities. Following a call for research proposals in July, 290 preliminary applications were received and the first successful projects were commissioned in December.

A new National Breast-feeding Working Group held three meetings during 1993. Its terms of reference are "to co-ordinate the next stages in a programme of action to promote and facilitate breast-feeding, building on the achievements of the Joint Breast-feeding Initiative", and its work will be co-ordinated with the United Nations UNICEF Baby Friendly Initiative.

References

1. Department of Health. The *Health of the Nation: a strategy for health in England*. London: HMSO, 1992 (Cm. 1986).
2. Department of Health. *The Nutrition Task Force Public Consultation on its Programme for Achieving the Health of the Nation Dietary Targets*. London: Department of Health, 1993.

(d)   Implementation

(i)   *NHS activities*

The first year of the *Health of the Nation* initiative[1] saw the NHS making major commitments to develop local action towards achieving the aims and specific targets of the strategy. During 1993, these commitments have been converted into action. In particular, the improving of public health through implementation of the Health of the Nation Strategy was identified as one of the top priorities for the NHS in its *Priorities and Planning Guidance 1994/95*[2], published in June. Plans to implement the strategy were produced by Regional Health Authorities (RHAs) in January, and set out details of how the strategy would be taken forward locally. RHAs and District Health Authorities (DHAs) established programmes of work to meet national targets, taking account of local needs, variations in health and activities already under way to promote health. This task involved local objective setting and negotiations between RHAs and DHAs on the balance to be struck between health promotion, treatment and care. Some RHAs have set additional targets and have used their local health strategy as the basis for local purchasing and health investment plans. The strategy's objectives have been reflected in corporate contracts, joint purchasing plans and service agreements as well as many varied local initiatives, including sexual health clinics for young people, health promotion programmes, and the creation of extra posts such as dietitians.

The NHS Management Executive supported the NHS in taking forward the strategy for health. The Chief Executive's Working Group on NHS Implementation has been charged with steering implementation of the strategy in and through the NHS, and key area handbooks[3,4,5,6,7] for managers and health professionals were published in January. The Health at Work in the NHS initiative, launched by the NHS Management Executive, continues to promote the importance of the NHS improving the health of its own staff and has produced the first of a series of good practice guides[8]. DH, in conjunction with the professions nationally, and local managers and clinicians, has explored ways to develop health promotion arrangements in primary care. The first *Targeting Practice* handbook[9] was published in September and describes the contribution of nurses, midwives and health visitors in each of the five key areas.

Research was commissioned to develop methods of setting and monitoring targets at local level, and a discussion paper setting out the main issues was published in July[10]. A series of meetings with RHAs in the Autumn led to an agreement to set regional targets, corresponding with those at national level, by the end of 1993. A network of regional *Health of the Nation* co-ordinators has met regularly with DH officials to exchange ideas and to identify ways to take the strategy forward, and a reference group was set up to develop guidance on health promotion in hospitals; a series of consultative workshops was held in the Autumn.

(ii)   Local health alliances

One of the central themes of the *Health of the Nation* initiative is the need to work together to achieve better health through 'health alliances'. Such alliances are not new, but the strategy for health emphasises the gains which can be made through such co-operation and has encouraged their further development. Local strategies for health have been jointly produced by health authorities, local authorities and a range of voluntary bodies working in partnership - such as the 'Partners for Health Alliance' in Brent, North West London, which includes Brent Council, the DHA and the local Family Health Services Authority (FHSA). Other alliances focus on more narrowly defined issues; for example, worshippers at a mosque in South London have arranged with local FHSAs to provide well-woman, family planning and cervical cytology services at the mosque.

To support the development of local health alliances, the handbook *Working Together for Better Health*[11] was published and more than 20,000 copies distributed in 1993. This booklet explains how health alliances can be set up and maintained, and sets out the advantages and benefits of working together, as well as being realistic about the difficulties and pitfalls. Evaluation of the impact of health alliances has not been forgotten. The Health Education Authority has funded a project to help to develop evaluation criteria, which should become available during 1994.

(iii)   Healthy settings

Seven 'healthy settings' - cities, schools, hospitals, the workplace, homes, the environment and prisons - were identified in the strategy for health[1]. Every individual spends at least part of their time in more than one of these settings, and the use of these settings helps to provide a focus for local action and may help with implementation of the strategy and the setting of local targets. The concept of healthy settings was explored at a conference held in November, where examples of good practice included Parrs Wood High School in Didsbury, Manchester, as an example of a health-promoting school where the whole curriculum reflects concerns for wider issues including health in the environment and the community; the Young Offenders Institution at Lancaster, a prison which aims to rehabilitate offenders, prevent suicides through an anti-bullying approach, and emphasises the dangers of drug misuse; and Kellogg's offices in

Manchester, a workplace which promotes healthy initiatives including a fitness centre induction training, and the availability of physical fitness tests for its workforce.

At a national level, further initiatives have been developed. The Prison Health Service is evaluating the impact of draft guidance on a wide variety of health promotion programmes issued to five establishments during 1993; a study of the mental health of unsentenced prisoners was started; fieldwork for a pilot study of anonymised HIV surveys in three prisons was completed and another pilot study of knowledge, attitudes and behaviour related to HIV infection and AIDS was started; and a survey of the physical health of male prisoners is planned for 1994. Our knowledge of the impact of the environment on health should be improved by the MRC's establishment of an Institute for the Environment and Health in Leicester, supported by funding from the Department of the Environment and DH (see page 165).

(iv)   Inter-Departmental co-operation

The strategy for health is not just a matter for DH and the NHS, but needs to be taken into account by every Government Department. A Cabinet Committee, which is chaired by the Lord President of the Council, co-ordinates the implementation, monitoring and development of the strategy across different Government Departments in England as well as co-ordinating efforts across the United Kingdom as a whole.

Many Government Departments and agencies have contributed to the development of the strategy through active participation in various Working Groups and Task Forces, and Ministers from three other Government Departments and the Lord President of the Council emphasised their commitment to it at a press conference on the publication of *One Year On*[12].

Government Departments are contributing to the success of the strategy within their own areas of responsibility. For instance, several have published advice about HIV/AIDS: the Home Office has developed educational packages for prisoners and prison officers; the Ministry of Defence provides education programmes for new recruits to the armed forces and those in service, including specific briefing for those posted overseas; and the Department of Employment and the Health and Safety Executive have produced a leaflet for employers on AIDS in the workplace.

References

1. Department of Health. *The Health of the Nation: a strategy for health in England.* London: HMSO, 1992 (Cm. 1986).
2. NHS Management Executive. *Priorities and Planning Guidance 1994/95.* Heywood (Lancashire): NHS Management Executive, 1993 (Executive Letter: EL(93)54).
3. Department of Health. *The Health of the Nation Key Area Handbook: coronary heart disease and stroke.* London: Department of Health, 1993.
4. Department of Health. *The Health of the Nation Key Area Handbook: cancers.* London: Department of Health, 1993.

5. Department of Health. *The Health of the Nation Key Area Handbook: mental illness.* London: Department of Health, 1993.
6. Department of Health. *The Health of the Nation Key Area Handbook: HIV/AIDS and sexual health.* London: Department of Health, 1993.
7. Department of Health. *The Health of the Nation Key Area Handbook: accidents.* London: Department of Health, 1993.
8. Health Education Authority. *Health at Work in the NHS: action pack.* London: Health Education Authority, 1992.
9. Department of Health. *Targeting Practice: the contribution of nurses, midwives and health visitors.* Heywood (Lancashire): Department of Health, 1993.
10. Department of Health. *Local Target Setting: a discussion paper.* London: Department of Health, 1993.
11. Department of Health. *Working Together for Better Health.* London: Department of Health, 1993.
12. Department of Health. *The Health of the Nation: one year on - a report on the progress of the Health of the Nation.* London: Department of Health, 1993.

(e)   The way ahead

The aims of the second year of the strategy are to build upon the momentum generated during the first year, and to focus on the development and provision of help for all those working in health promotion.

Following the publication of the handbook *Working Together for Better Health*[1], the Alliances subgroup of the Wider Health Working Group is developing an awards scheme to encourage partnerships between organisations outside the health service to be set up to improve the health of local populations. The scheme will be launched in the Summer of 1994, with the first awards to be presented in the following year.

Reference

1. Department of Health. *Working Together for Better Health.* London: Department of Health, 1993.

CHAPTER 4

THE HEALTH OF ADOLESCENTS

Introduction

Recent Reports have looked in detail at the health of different sections of the population, such as children[1], women of reproductive age and the menopause[2], people in later life[3], black and ethnic minorities[4] and men[5]. This chapter looks at the health of adolescents, defined as young people aged from 10-19 years[6]; however, because this definition is not universally applied, age ranges are included for specific data where appropriate.

Adolescence is the transitional phase between childhood and adulthood, characterised by experimentation and rapid change. It is a key time for learning, mainly by exploration of new ideas and behaviours, for consolidating health-related values, attitudes, and lifestyles[7], and for making decisions about various behaviours which have important consequences for future health. The purpose of adolescent health care is to support this process and to enable young people to become healthy and competent adults[8].

Passing through the inter-related stages of cognitive, social, emotional and physical development of adolescence requires considerable adaptation, and failure to negotiate these developmental hurdles successfully may have far-reaching consequences[9]. Cultural expectations exert further pressures[10].

Recent social and legal changes, along with advances in health care, have brought additional influences to bear. For example, a rise in unemployment among school-leavers, a shortage of alternative housing and time spent in full-time education all lengthen the period of dependency on parents[11]. Young people have acquired rights in law to self-determination[12], and those with life-threatening illnesses, previously fatal in childhood, may now survive and require continuing care into adolescence and young adulthood[11]. Young people are adopting patterns of risk behaviour at an earlier age[11], and in choosing such lifestyles may appear heedless of the health consequences of, for example, cigarette smoking, alcohol or sexual activity[7].

Between 1982 and 1992, the total number of adolescents in England has fallen by 21.7% to less than six million, while the total population rose by 3.4% to just over 48 million. Thus the proportion of adolescents has fallen from 16% of the total population in 1982 to only 12.1% in 1992. However, this trend will reverse over the next 20 years, with forecasts of an increase of over 10% (to 6.5 million) in the adolescent population between 1992 and 2012, compared with a near 7% increase in the total population. These changes are shown in Table 4.1 and Figures 4.1 and 4.2.

Table 4.1: *Population estimates and projections, England, 1982-2012*

Population in thousands	1982	1992	2002 projections	2012 projections	% change 1982-1992	% change 1992-2002	% change 2002-2012
Total population aged 10-19 years	7497	5872	6400	6481	-21.7	9.0	1.3
Male population aged 10-19 years	3853	3021	3289	3324	-21.6	8.9	1.0
Female population aged 10-19 years	3644	2852	3110	3157	-21.7	9.1	1.5
Total population all ages	46807	48378	50194	51566	3.4	3.8	2.7
Male population all ages	22788	23688	24798	25623	3.9	4.7	3.3
Female population all ages	24020	24691	25396	25942	2.8	2.9	2.2
Population 10-19 years as % of total population all ages	16.0	12.1	12.8	12.6			
Males 10-19 years as % of total male population all ages	16.9	12.8	13.3	13.0			
Females 10-19 years as % of total female population all ages	15.2	11.5	12.2	12.2			

Note: All figures are independently rounded.

Source: OPCS for 1982 and 1992 population estimates; Government Actuary's Department (GAD) for 2002 and 2012 population projections

References

1. Department of Health. *On the State of the Public Health: the annual report of the Chief Medical Officer of the Department of Health for the year 1988.* London: HMSO, 1989; 65.
2. Department of Health. *On the State of the Public Health: the annual report of the Chief Medical Officer of the Department of Health for the year 1989.* London: HMSO, 1990; 54.
3. Department of Health. *On the State of the Public Health: the annual report of the Chief Medical Officer of the Department of Health for the year 1990.* London: HMSO, 1991; 68.
4. Department of Health. *On the State of the Public Health: the annual report of the Chief Medical Officer of the Department of Health for the year 1991.* London: HMSO, 1992; 54.
5. Department of Health. *On the State of the Public Health: the annual report of the Chief Medical Officer of the Department of Health for the year 1992.* London: HMSO, 1993; 79.
6. World Health Organization. PB/90-91. Geneva: WHO, 1988.
7. Hurrelmann K, Losel F, eds. *Health hazards in adolescence.* Berlin: Walter de Gruyter, 1990.
8. Strasburger VC, Brown RT. *Adolescent medicine: a practical guide.* Boston: Little, Brown, 1991.
9. Kaufman K, Brown R, Graves K, Henderson P, Revolinski M. What, Me Worry? A survey of adolescents' concerns. *Clin Pediatr* 1993; **32**: 8-14.
10. Brannen J, Dodd K, Oakley A, Storey P. *Young people, health and family life.* Buckingham: Open University Press (in press).
11. Woodroffe C, Glickman M, Barber M, Power C. *Children, Teenagers and Health. The key data.* Oxford: Oxford University Press, 1991.
12. *Children Act 1989.* London: HMSO, 1989.

Figure 4.1: *Population estimates and projections, England, 1982-2012*

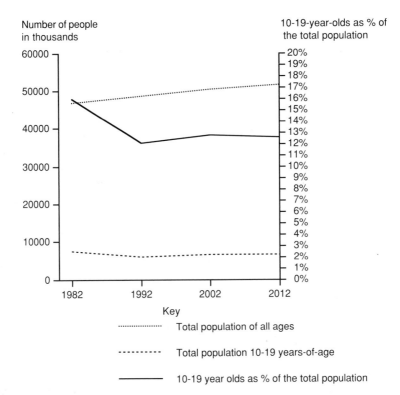

Source: 1982 and 1992 population figures from OPCS; projections from GAD

Figure 4.2: *Population estimates and projections, England, 1982-2012*

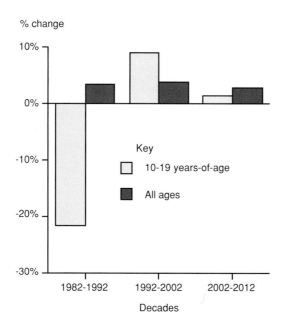

Source: OPCS for 1982 and 1992 estimates; GAD for 2002 and 2012 projections

(a)   Mortality

The main causes of death among young adolescents in England and Wales in 1982 and 1992 are shown in Table 4.2 and Figure 4.3. Over half the total deaths in 1992 were due to injury and poisoning, accounting for 24 deaths per 100,000 adolescent population in males and 9 deaths per 100,000 in females. Neoplasms were the second largest cause, representing 13% of deaths among males (or 5 deaths per 100,000) and 16% among females (or 3 deaths per 100,000) in 1992. The third commonest cause of death was diseases of the nervous system (3 and 2 deaths per 100,000 population, respectively, for males and females), the major causes including epilepsy and, in males, muscular dystrophies. Respiratory diseases were the fourth biggest killer in 1982, but had fallen by 1992 to less than 1 death per 100,000 population for both sexes, and were no longer a major cause of death in this age-group.

Between 1982 and 1992, the overall number of deaths among adolescents fell by 42% among males and 33% among females, corresponding to a fall in the underlying death rate of 26% in males and 14% in females. Most causes of death showed a reduction during this period - the only notable exception was "mental disorders", although only relatively small numbers were involved (see Figure 4.4). Over the same period the death rates in most other age-groups also fell. In comparison with other countries, overall death rates among children and young adolescents aged 5-14 years in England and Wales are low (see Table 4.3 and Figure 4.5).

Table 4.2: *Mortality in adolescents aged 10-19 years, England and Wales, 1982-92*

Cause of death	Number of deaths 1982		1992		Percentage change 1982-92		Death rates per 100,000 population 1982		1992		Percentage change in death rates, 1982-92	
	Males	Females	Males	Females	Males %	Females %	Males	Females	Males	Females	Males %	Females %
Infectious and parasitic	34	21	29	28	-14.7	33.3	0.88	0.58	0.96	0.98	8.78	70.36
Neoplasms	259	165	165	98	-36.3	-40.6	6.72	4.53	5.46	3.44	-18.75	-24.11
Endocrine and nutritional	41	32	33	24	-19.5	-25.0	1.06	0.88	1.09	0.84	2.65	-4.17
Diseases of blood	11	11	6	5	-45.5	-54.5	0.29	0.30	0.20	0.18	-30.43	-41.92
Mental disorders	20	9	53	14	165.0	55.6	0.52	0.25	1.75	0.49	237.98	98.75
Nervous system	126	74	105	56	-16.7	-24.3	3.27	2.03	3.48	1.96	6.28	-3.31
Circulatory	72	50	51	39	-29.2	-22.0	1.87	1.37	1.69	1.37	-9.66	-0.34
Respiratory system	111	60	29	21	-73.9	-65.0	2.88	1.65	0.96	0.74	-66.68	-55.28
Digestive	24	14	7	9	-70.8	-35.7	0.62	0.38	0.23	0.32	-62.80	-17.86
Genito-urinary	10	11	4	2	-60.0	-81.8	0.26	0.30	0.13	0.07	-48.98	-76.77
Musculo-skeletal system	5	12	2	12	-60.0	0.0	0.13	0.33	0.07	0.42	-48.98	27.77
Congenital	94	56	40	53	-57.4	-5.4	2.44	1.54	1.32	1.86	-45.73	20.93
Injury and poisoning	1405	415	759	262	-46.0	-36.9	36.47	11.39	25.12	9.19	-31.10	-19.34
Other	3	11	8	8	166.7	-27.3	0.08	0.30	0.26	0.28	240.11	-7.08
Total	2215	941	1291	631	-41.7	-32.9	57.49	25.82	42.73	22.12	-25.66	-14.32

Source: OPCS DH2 nos. 9 and 19, Table 2

Figure 4.3: *Mortality in adolescents by cause of death, England and Wales, 1992*

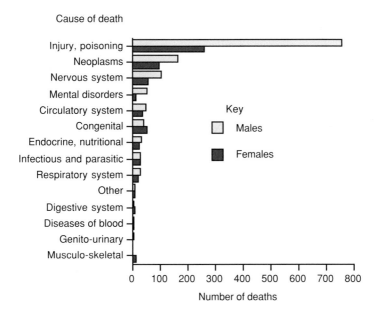

Source: OPCS DH2 nos. 9 and 19, Table 2

Figure 4.4: *Mortality in adolescents, England and Wales (percentage change 1982-92)*

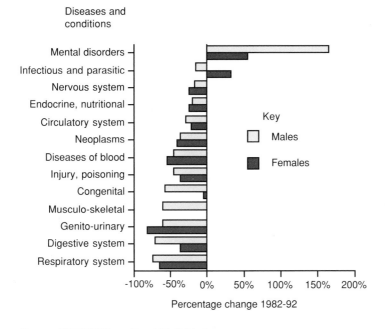

Source: OPCS DH2 nos. 9 and 19, Table 2

Figure 4.5: *Mortality from all causes at age 5-14 years, by country, 1990-92*

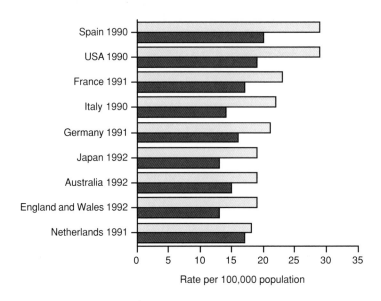

Table 4.3: *Mortality from all causes at age 5-14 years, by country, 1990-92*

			Deaths per 100,000 population	
Country	Year		Males	Females
USA	1990		29	19
Spain	1990		29	20
Australia	1992		19	15
France	1991		23	17
Germany	1991		21	16
Italy	1990		22	14
England & Wales	1992		19	13
Netherlands	1991		18	17
Japan	1992		19	13

Source: WHO Annual 1993

(b)   Morbidity

Studies of adolescent mobidity are few and routine statistics do not provide specific adolescent disease profiles. Adolescents are usually regarded as healthy beings "making few demands on medical resources and showing little interest in their own health"[1], but studies indicate more illness and higher use of health services than this view would support[1]. Self-reported illness is recorded in the General Household Survey (GHS), which provides a measure of individuals' perception of health. In common with all other age-groups, the proportion of 5-

15-year-olds reporting long-standing illness has shown a general increase (with some fluctuations) over the past 13 years. Based on preliminary figures from the 1992 GHS, self-reported illness rose from 14% to 19% among males and from 10% to 18% among females between 1979 and 1992, although there was a slight reduction in 5-15-year-olds reporting restricted activity in the two weeks before the survey; the figures show slight year-on-year fluctuations (see Table 4.4 and Figure 4.6).

In 1985, a questionnaire survey of 14-16-year-olds in Oxford showed that 92% felt their health was good or fair and 7% thought it excellent; nevertheless, at the time of the survey, 45% reported some concurrent health problem - mostly coughs and colds - and 37% had seen their general practitioner (GP) in the previous three months, again for common ailments. In the four weeks before the survey, 37% had time off school with gastro-intestinal problems or coughs and colds and 70% had taken medicines, mainly for headaches and coughs and colds[1].

GP consultations provide an indication of morbidity in the population. Data recorded in the GHS indicate that young people consult their GP three to four times a year on average. Further information is available from surveys of Morbidity Statistics from General Practice[2,3]. Respiratory tract diseases are the major cause of consultation in those aged 5-15 and 16-24 years. Both age-groups showed an increase in overall patient consulting rates between 1981-82 and 1991-92 from 669 to 723 per 1,000 person-years at risk for those aged 5-14/15 years, and from 705 to 757 per 1,000 person-years at risk in those aged 15/16-24

Figure 4.6: *Trends in self-reported sickness in persons aged 5-15 years, Great Britain, 1979-92*

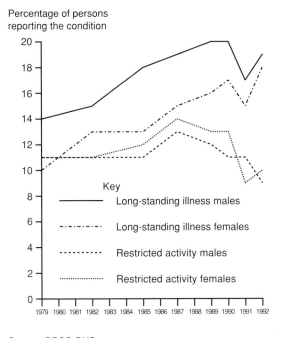

Percentage of persons
reporting the condition

Key

——————— Long-standing illness males

–·–·–·–·– Long-standing illness females

- - - - - - - - Restricted activity males

···················· Restricted activity females

Source: OPCS GHS

Table 4.4: Trends in self-reported sickness in persons aged 5-15 years (percentage of persons reporting long-standing illness or restricted activity), Great Britain, 1979-92

	1979	1980	1981	1982	1983	1984	1985	1986	1987	1988	1989	1990	1991	1992
Long-standing illness														
Males	14	16	17	15	17	18	18	20	19	21	20	20	17	19
Females	10	11	13	13	13	15	13	15	15	16	16	17	15	18
Restricted activity														
Males	11	13	12	11	12	11	11	13	13	11	12	11	11	9
Females	11	13	11	11	11	12	12	11	14	11	13	13	9	10

Source: OPCS, GHS

years (see Table 4.5 and Figure 4.7; different age bands were used between 1981-82 and 1991-92, and all comparisons should be treated with caution because of changes in survey conditions and methods). These patient consulting rates are broadly similar to those for adults aged 25-64 years, but are lower than those for adults aged 65 years and over (see Table 4.6 and Figure 4.8).

The GHS also indicates use of other National Health Service (NHS) facilities. Reported attendances at outpatient or accident and emergency departments increased slightly between 1979 and 1992, from 10% to 12% of males and from 8% to 10% of females aged 5-15 years. The proportion of 5-15-year-olds reporting inpatient stays is the same in 1992 as in 1987.

Hospital admission rates are lower at 10-14 years and 15-19 years than for most 5-year age-groups[4] (see Table 4.7 and Figure 4.9). Table 4.8 and Figure 4.10 show hospital inpatient cases by specialty for 5-14-year-olds: injury and poisoning dominate with rates of 16.6 per 1,000 population for males and 10 per 1,000 population for females, closely followed by respiratory and nervous system disorders[5].

The Oxford Unit of Health Care Epidemiology, with information from 1979-86, has shown that admissions to hospital for adolescents are more likely to be surgical than medical. At 10 years-of-age, 20% of male admissions in the Oxford region[6] were for trauma and orthopaedics, increasing to 40% of male admissions at 16 years. At 10 years-of-age, female admission rates for trauma and orthopaedics are similar to those for males, but by 16 years less than half as

Figure 4.7: *Patient consulting rates aged 5-15 and 16-24 years, England and Wales, 1991-92*

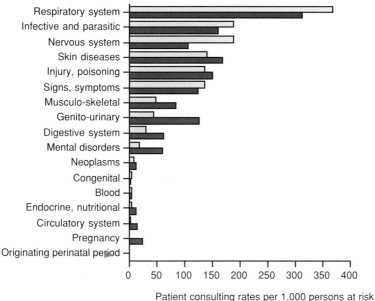

Patient consulting rates per 1,000 persons at risk

Table 4.5: GP consultations: patient consulting rates per 1,000 person-years at risk, England and Wales, 1981-82 and 1991-92

	1981-82		1991-92		Percentage change 1981-82 to 1991-92	
	Age 5-14 years	Age 15-24 years	Age 5-15 years	Age 16-24 years	Age 5-14/15 years	Age 15/16-24 years
All diseases	668.6	705.4	723.4	757.2	8	7
Infective and parasitic	175.9	129.7	188.8	160.2	7	24
Neoplasms	2.9	5.2	8.8	13.3	203	156
Endocrine, nutritional	4.8	16.3	4.3	12.0	-10	-26
Blood	2.9	4.5	5.6	5.5	93	22
Mental disorders	17.2	63.7	19.4	61.1	13	-4
Nervous system	164.0	94.9	188.1	106.7	15	12
Circulatory system	1.4	12.4	2.6	14.6	86	18
Respiratory system	341.4	259.4	368.0	312.0	8	20
Digestive system	32.0	55.2	30.6	63.2	-4	14
Genito-urinary	29.8	111.8	45.3	127.9	52	14
Pregnancy	0.2	20.6	0.5	24.7	150	20
Skin diseases	114.1	146.8	141.8	169.7	24	16
Musculo-skeletal	41.3	82.0	48.9	84.2	18	3
Congenital	4.6	1.8	5.9	3.3	28	83
Originating perinatal period	0.1	0.0	0.0	0.2	n/a	n/a
Signs, symptons	149.7	134.3	136.3	124.6	-9	-7
Injury, poisoning	117.6	134.8	137.5	151.8	17	13

Note: Different age bands were used in 1981-82 and 1991-92.

Source: OPCS MSGP-3, 1981-82 & MSGP-4, 1991-92

Table 4.6: *Consultations in general practice: patient consulting rates for all diseases at per 1,000 person-years at risk, England and Wales, 1981-82 and 1991-92*

1981-82		1991-92	
Age-group	Rate	Age-group	Rate
5-14 years	668.6	5-15 years	723.4
15-24 years	705.4	16-24 years	757.2
25-44 years	678.8	25-44 years	735.7
45-64 years	674.9	45-64 years	761.0
65-74 years	738.8	65-74 years	827.1
75+ years	789.0	75-84 years	905.0
		85+ years	919.3

Note: Different age bands were used in 1981/82 and 1991/92.

Source: OPCS MSGP-3 and MSGP-4

Figure 4.8: *Consultations in general practice: patient consulting rates for all diseases per 1,000 person-years at risk, England and Wales, 1981-82 and 1991-92*

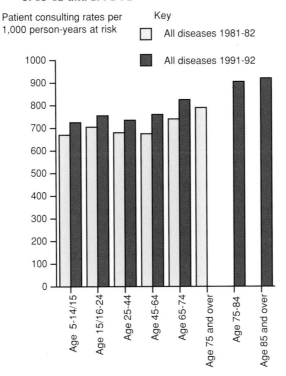

Note: Different age bands were used in 1981-82 and 1991-92.

Source: OPCS MSGP-3 and MSGP-4

Table 4.7: Discharge rates from hospital per 10,000 population aged 0-4 to 85+ years, England , 1985

	All ages	0-4 years	5-9 years	10-14 years	15-19 years	20-24 years	25-29 years	30-34 years	35-39 years	40-44 years	45-49 years	50-54 years	55-59 years	60-64 years	65-69 years	70-74 years	75-79 years	80-84 years	85 years +
Total	1074.3	1500.6	723.2	534.5	649.5	728.1	753.0	759.9	735.4	772.3	864.2	945.8	1078.3	1297.0	1562.1	2000.4	2539.2	3168.6	4001.7
Male	1032.1	1757.3	855.6	596.5	571.8	576.1	541.7	539.1	531.8	593.6	746.4	923.7	1175.0	1498.0	1846.6	2427.8	3146.9	3757.0	4860.8
Female	1114.5	1230.7	583.4	468.9	731.3	884.8	968.5	984.5	939.6	954.0	983.1	967.9	984.9	1113.8	1324.6	1684.7	2166.1	2893.0	3741.4

Source: Hospital Inpatient Enquiry 1985

Figure 4.9: *Discharge rates from hospital per 10,000 population, England, 1985*

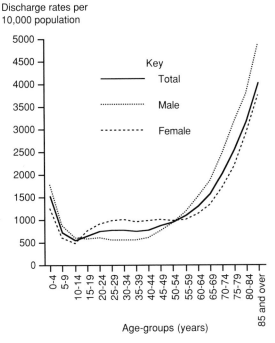

Source: Hospital Inpatient Enquiry 1985

many females are admitted compared with males. Throughout adolescence, by far the most common cause of male admission is head injury and the second commonest cause is 'open wounds'[6]; admission rates relate to the degree of trauma - most fractures, unlike head injuries, tend to be treated on an outpatient basis. Head injuries also account for a high number of hospital bed-days, even though many are short admissions for observation[7]. The most common reason for hospital admission for young women from the ages of 15-16 years is termination of pregnancy or childbirth[6]. For adolescents admitted to hospital, long stays for accidents are associated with fractured femur and burns[7]. Some of the most common individual reasons for admission are behavioural disorders rather than disease processes[7].

References

1. Macfarlane A, McPherson A, McPherson K, Ahmed L. Teenagers and their health. *Arch Dis Childh* 1987; **62**: 1125-9.
2. Office of Population Censuses and Surveys. *Morbidity Statistics from General Practice 1981-82*. London: HMSO, 1984 (MB5 No.1).
3. Office of Population Censuses and Surveys. *Morbidity Statistics from General Practice 1991-92*. London: HMSO (in press).
4. Department of Health and Social Security, Office of Population Censuses and Surveys. *Hospital inpatient enquiry: summary tables-1985*. London: HMSO, 1987.
5. Department of Health. *Hospital Episode Statistics 1989/90. Volume 1*. London: Department of Health, 1993.
6. Henderson J, Goldacre M, Yeates D. Use of hospital in patient care in adolescence. *Arch Dis Childh* 1993; **69**: 559-63.
7. Henderson J, Goldacre M, Fairweather J, Marcovitch H. Conditions accounting for substantial time spent in hospital in childhood aged 1-14 years. Arch Dis Childh 1992; **67**: 83-6.

Table 4.8: *Hospital inpatient cases: ordinary admissions plus day cases aged 5-14 years per 1,000 population, England 1990-91*

	Total cases		Rate per 1,000	
	Males	Females	Males	Females
All diagnoses	252543	183020	84.2	64.6
Infective and parasitic	5987	5312	2.0	1.9
Neoplasms	6796	6992	2.3	2.5
Endocrine, nutritional	3531	3831	1.2	1.4
Blood	4404	4299	1.5	1.5
Mental disorders	7442	7042	2.5	2.5
Nervous system	36394	27346	12.1	9.7
Circulatory system	753	648	0.3	0.2
Respiratory system	47018	31674	15.7	11.2
Digestive system	25333	23974	8.4	8.5
Genito-urinary	22682	1772	7.6	0.6
Pregnancy	0	1075	0.0	0.4
Skin diseases	5253	4139	1.8	1.5
Musculo-skeletal	8097	8616	2.7	3.0
Congenital	15355	7569	5.1	2.7
Originating perinatal period	119	81	0.0	0.0
Signs, symptoms	18723	18310	6.2	6.5
Injury, poisoning	44656	30340	14.9	10.7

Source: HES 1990-91 tables 3.1, 3.2

Figure 4.10: *Hospital inpatient cases (day cases and ordinary admissions) aged 5-14 years, England, 1989-90*

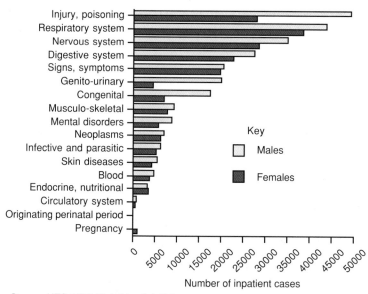

Source: HES 1989-90, tables 3.1, 3.2

88

(c) Specific conditions

(i) Injury

Road traffic accidents account for three-quarters of all accidental deaths in the 15-24 years age-group[1] and alcohol-related road fatalities are particularly common among young people[2]. Accidents in the home account for 12% of injuries in the 15-24 years age-group[1], while sporting injuries in young people account for 5-10% of all attendances to accident and emergency departments[3]. Occupational accidents are also an important cause of morbidity and mortality in young people, the most common causes of fatality involving falling, being struck by a moving object and mechanical strangulation[4].

(ii) Cancer

About 900 new cases of cancer are reported annually in people aged 10-19 years in England and Wales. Hodgkin's disease and other lymphomas account for 22% of cases, followed by leukaemias and brain tumours at 16% and 14%, respectively. Gonadal tumours account for 9% of cases in both sexes combined, with a 6% incidence of testicular tumours in boys (see Table 4.9 and Figure 4.11).

(iii) Diabetes mellitus

Diabetes mellitus affects 1-2% of the population, although it is particularly prevalent among Asians and Afro-Caribbeans. In adolescents, the prevalence of clinically diagnosed diabetes mellitus has been estimated to be about 2 per 1,000 population[5]. Diabetes mellitus accounts for about 0.6% of hospital episodes in 5-14-year-olds but causes only a very small number of deaths (6 deaths in 1992).

(iv) Asthma

Of children with persistent symptoms of asthma at the age of 7 years, 80% still have symptoms in adolescence; girls appear to do less well than boys[6]. A recent Australian survey[7] has shown that in mid-adolescence smoking is more common among those with asthma symptoms than those without.

The 1991 National Asthma Survey (unpublished data) showed a profile of symptom severity and distribution of care similar to that of the population at all ages. Asthma is one of the commonest conditions in childhood and adolescence, with long hospital stays and large numbers of bed days used[8]. GP consultations have risen markedly over the last 10 years, but comparisons may be affected by improved diagnosis. Asthma[9], like other chronic physical illnesses in young people[10], has a higher incidence of associated mental health problems than is to be found in the general child population.

Table 4.9: Cancer registrations in adolescents, England and Wales, 1988

	ICD9 code	Males	%	Females	%	Persons	%
All malignant neoplasms	140-208	538		381		919	
Bone	170	55	10	30	8	85	9
Soft tissue	171	21	4	22	6	43	5
Malignant melanoma	172	16	3	25	7	41	4
Other skin	173	28	5	21	6	49	5
Ovary	183			28	7	28	3
Testis	186	55				55	6
Brain	191	83	15	42	11	125	14
Hodgkin's	201	65	12	60	16	125	14
Lymphoid	202	53	10	23	6	76	8
All leukaemias	204-208	98	18	46	12	144	16
Other		64	12	84	22	148	16

Source: OPCS MB 1 No. 21

Figure 4.11: *Cancer registrations in adolescents, England and Wales, 1988*

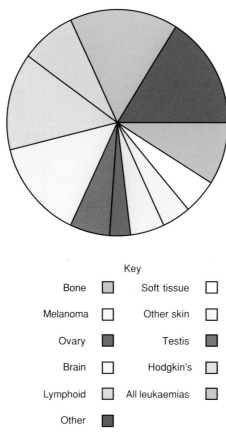

Key

Bone	■	Soft tissue	□
Melanoma	□	Other skin	□
Ovary	■	Testis	■
Brain	□	Hodgkin's	■
Lymphoid	■	All leukaemias	■
Other	■		

Source: OPCS MB1 No. 21

(v)   Sexually transmitted diseases

Table 4.10 shows cumulative AIDS case reports and HIV infection diagnoses in adolescents grouped by sex and exposure category. At the end of 1993, AIDS had been notified in 48 and HIV infection in 498 adolescent males, with 6 AIDS cases and 72 HIV infections in adolescent females.

Other sexually transmitted diseases (STDs) become increasingly prominent in later adolescence, particularly in females. For example, about one-third of reports of post-pubertal uncomplicated gonorrhoea diagnosed in females are in

Table 4.10: *AIDS cases and HIV infections diagnosed in adolescents to end December 1993*

How persons probably acquired the virus	AIDS cases		HIV infections	
	Male	Female	Male	Female
Sexual intercourse				
between men	9*	-	203	-
between men and women	2	5	10	47
Injecting drug use (IDU)	-	-	17	14
Blood				
Blood factor (eg for haemophilia)	35		244	-
Blood tissue transfer (eg transfusion)	2	1	16	7
Not known	-	-	8	4
Total	48	6	498	72

*Includes 1 report of transmission through IDU or sex between men.
Source: CDSC

Table 4.11: *Number of new cases seen in NHS genito-urinary medicine clinics, England, 1992*

Condition	Sex	Under 16 years	16-19 years	All ages	Estimated median age (years)	Percentage of cases in those aged 19 years and under
Infectious syphilis	M	0	4	228	34	1.8
	F	3	15	110	27	16.4
Post-pubertal uncomplicated gonorrhoea	M	43	834	7691	26	11.4
	F	116	1370	4401	22	33.8
Post-pubertal uncomplicated chlamydia	M	27	1235	13089	25	9.6
	F	271	4209	15309	22	29.3
Herpes simplex - first attack	M	17	331	6140	29	5.7
	F	72	1333	7877	24	17.8
Wart virus infection - first attack	M	94	2226	27169	25	8.5
	F	340	6269	23955	22	27.6

M = male, F = female.

Source: DH, Form KC60 returns

Figure 4.12: *New cases seen in NHS genito-urinary medicine clinics by age (years) and sex, England, 1992*

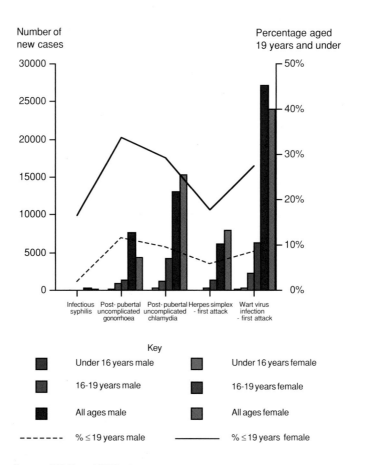

Source: DH, Form KC60 returns

those aged 19 years and younger, and numbers of cases of other STDs in those aged 19 years or younger are significantly higher in females than in males (see Table 4.11 and Figure 4.12). These figures show the need for continuing safer sex advice focused on young people.

(vi)   Dental health

The dental health of adolescents has shown a remarkable improvement, particularly over the last ten years. From 1983 to 1993, the proportion of 15-year-olds with active, untreated tooth decay fell from 42% to 30%, or approximately 160,000 young people, and the proportion free from caries increased five-fold, from 8% to 40%. The proportion with fillings is now 48% compared with 85% in 1983, and only 6% have had teeth extracted because of decay compared with 21% in 1983.

There are, however, substantial regional and ethnic variations. Some young ethnic groups, residing in deprived social areas, have poorer oral hygiene than others and the widespread use of tobacco chewing with betel-quid by some young women has carcinogenic potential for the future[11]. Monitoring and oral health promotion for the at-risk indigenous and ethnic population is a priority.

References

1. Department of Health. *The Health of the Nation Key Area Handbook: accidents.* London: Department of Health, 1993.
2. Department of Transport. *Road Accidents in Great Britain in 1992.* London: HMSO, 1993.
3. Medical Royal Colleges of the UK. *Strategies for Accident Prevention: report of the Colloquium of the Medical Royal Colleges of the UK.* London: Department of Health and Social Security, 1988.
4. Office of Population Censuses and Surveys. *Mortality Statistics: injury and poisoning.* London: HMSO, 1991.
5. Stevens A, Raftery J, eds. *Health Care Needs Assessment: the epidemiologically based needs assessment reviews: volume 1.* Southampton: Wessex Institute of Public Health Medicine, 1993.
6. Martin AL, Martin AJ, McLennan LA, Landau LI, Phelan PD. The natural history of childhood asthma to adult life. *BMJ* 1980; **i:** 1397-400.
7. Forero R, Bauman A, Young L, Larkin P. Asthma prevalence and management of Australian adolescents: results from the community surveys. *J Adolescent Health* 1992; **13:** 707-12.
8. Henderson J, Goldacre M, Fairweather J, Marcovitch H. Conditions accounting for substantial time spent in hospital in childhood aged 1-14 years. *Arch Dis Childh* 1992; **67:** 83-6.
9. Miller BD. Depression and asthma: a potentially lethal mixture. *J Allergy Clin Immunol* 1987; **80:** 48.
10. Orr DP, Weller SC, Satterwhite B, Pless IB. Psychosocial implications of chronic disease in adolescence. *J Pediatr* 1984; **104:** 152-7.
11. Johnson NW, Warnakulasuriya KAAS. Epidemiology and aetiology of oral cancer in the United Kingdom. *Commun Dent Health* 1993: **10 (Suppl 1):** 13-29.

(d)   Lifestyle and health

Health-related lifestyle factors play a major part in the aetiology of cardiovascular and respiratory disease, some cancers and other conditions which account for much of the burden of mortality and morbidity in later life. The establishment of a healthy lifestyle during adolescence has wide-ranging benefits: in the short term, a healthy lifestyle encourages optimum growth and resistance to physical and emotional ill-health; in the long term, the maintenance of a healthy lifestyle in adulthood is more likely if established during childhood[1]. For example, most adult smokers start smoking as teenagers[2].

Recent evidence indicates that class variations are much less pronounced in adolescence than in earlier or later life[3]. Between the ages of 10 and 14 years, social class gradients of all causes of mortality are narrower than at any other time[4]. In the 12-19 years age-group, rates of chronic illness show little or no variation among social class groups in any one-year age subgroup[3,4]. This is perhaps not surprising given that adolescence is biologically a less vulnerable time of life, and mortality and morbidity indicators less sensitive to variations among social groups. Other more specific health indices may provide a different picture. The importance of recognising cultural differences and orientating services to multicultural needs is becoming increasingly recognised[5,6].

The Health of the Nation key areas relating to physical activity, diet and nutrition, smoking and alcohol misuse are particularly relevant to adolescent health.

(i)   *Physical activity*

There is concern about the low levels of physical activity in young people under 16 years-of-age, especially girls who take less physical activity than women aged 16-45 years. Not only do fewer young people participate in sport, but fewer children now walk to school (62% in 1990, compared with 81% in 1970) and only 2% cycle to school[7]. However, a recent local survey of 14-year-olds showed 86% of boys and 81% girls claimed to take some form of regular exercise[8].

(ii)   *Diet and nutrition*

There is little information on the diet and nutrition of adolescents. A 1983 survey[9] examined the diets and nutrient intakes of a representative sample of British schoolchildren aged 14-15 years. Patterns were similar to those of adults, with about 38% of energy derived from fat, mainly from chips and milk, compared with the 35% recommended.

In girls, intakes of calcium, iron and riboflavin were lower than recommended[9]. There is more recent evidence for low iron stores in some groups of adolescent girls[10]. Low iron status and low calcium intake may be important for psychomotor and bone development, respectively[11,12].

Dietary intake data collected between April 1986 and July 1987 from a national sample of 16-17-year-olds in the follow-up of the 1970 longitudinal birth cohort study[13] showed that intakes of fats and extrinsic sugars exceeded Department of Health (DH) recommendations[14] and intakes of intrinsic sugars, milk sugars and starch and non-starch polysaccharides were lower.

(iii)   *Smoking*

Adult smoking prevalence continues to fall, but 1992 figures for cigarette smoking among 11-15-year-olds are virtually unchanged since 1986 at 10%. Although efforts will continue to reach young people through health education programmes, family example is an important factor in reducing teenage smoking[2]. Children of non-smoking parents are two-and-a-half times less likely to smoke than children whose parents smoke, and children are seven times less likely to smoke if they perceive strong parental disapproval[15]. The influence of siblings is also important[16]. Health education campaigns aimed at adults are being broadened to involve parents in tackling this problem.

(iv)   *Alcohol misuse*

From a very early age, young people develop a sophisticated awareness of alcohol and drinking behaviour. It appears that regular drinking, that is at least once a week, often begins at an early age and that weekly consumption in 14-15-year-olds is increasing[17,18]. Recent surveys show that 20% of 9-15-year-olds have had their first alcoholic drink by the age of 8 years, and 89% by 13 years[17].

Twelve per cent of 11-15-year-olds are regular drinkers[17,18], and young people are also at risk for drunkenness offences and related criminal behaviour[19].

The recommended sensible drinking limits for adults may be less applicable for young people and the proportion drinking in excess of them gives cause for concern. A Health Education Authority survey in 1992 showed that, among 11-15-year-olds who drank in the preceding week, 5% of girls exceeded the adult sensible limit of 14 units and 3% of boys exceeded the adult sensible limit of 21 units - the equivalent of 35,000 young people in England[17].

(v) Substance misuse

A wide range of drugs may be readily available to young people, but unlike alcohol and tobacco, the vast majority of young people never try a drug, and even fewer experiment with drugs or develop a serious drug problem[20].

A recent survey of male and female schoolchildren aged 9-15 years in England found that, by the age of 15 years, 16% of boys and 14% of girls, or approximately 7,500 each, had tried cannabis; 5% and 2%, respectively, had used lysergic acid diethylamide (LSD); 4% and 2%, respectively, amphetamines and solvents; and 3% and 1%, respectively, tranquillisers and ecstasy. Heroin, cocaine and crack had each been tried by 1%, or 500 each, of 15-year-old boys or girls[17].

Solvent misuse peaks at about the age of 15 years so that 2% of 15-year-olds reported currently using solvents and 9% reported using them in the past[18]. DH recognises the importance of health education in this field and in 1993 funded a media campaign aimed particularly at providing information and support for parents[21].

(vi) Sexual behaviour

Although the physical complications of adolescent pregnancy are only a little higher than in more mature women, there are major social consequences of a childhood and education cut short by the demands of motherhood. Alternatively, there is the emotional distress of abortion, resorted to by around half the girls who become pregnant before the age of 16 years. Of those girls who give birth, registration data indicate that most are not able to share the upbringing of the child with its father.

Over the past 10 years, adolescent conception rates have shown a small rise, but they dropped in the latest year for which statistics are available (see Figure 4.13). The rate in that year (1991), for girls aged 13-15 years, was 9.3 per 1,000, a fall of 8% on 1990. Rates are highest in areas of social deprivation.

Puberty brings powerful sexual feelings. By the age of 16 years, around a quarter of boys and a fifth of girls in Britain have experienced sexual intercourse[22]. Some girls see childbearing as the way to a more adult status[23].

Risk-taking and experimentation are significant features of adolescent behaviour[24] and sexual intercourse is no exception. Adolescents lack experience in handling personal relationships, and sexual intercourse may some times be perceived as the only way to maintain a close friendship. Lack of knowledge about, and ready access to, contraception can lead to unwanted pregnancy[25]: only around half of adolescents use contraceptives at first intercourse[22]. Other risk-related behaviour can be a factor in teenage conception, in particular the loss of inhibitions resulting from drug abuse or excess alcohol intake.

In the Netherlands, intervention halved the teenage conception rate through sex education programmes that covered the handling of relationships, information on contraception and accepted the reality of teenage sexuality. There adolescents have ready access to confidential counselling and contraception from general practitioners[26,27]. Research suggests that there is considerable unmet need for adolescents to discuss sexual development, sexually transmitted diseases and contraception[28], and in England services for teenagers are being improved[29] to help to remedy this shortfall. However, a study in Wessex found that 75% of adolescents aged under 16 years feared that their GP would not preserve confidentiality regarding requests for contraceptive services[30]. Guidance on confidentiality has been issued by the BMA in conjunction with other bodies[31].

Figure 4.13: *Conception rates for teenage females, England and Wales, 1969-91*

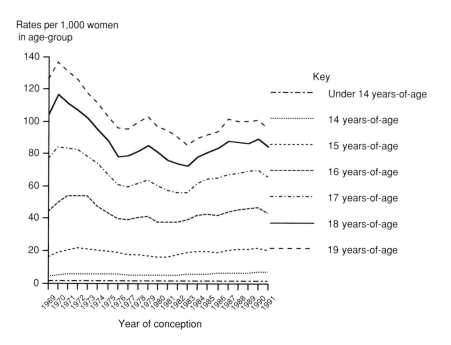

Source: OPCS birth statistics FM1 and *Population Trends* 73

98

(vii)   Mental health

Adolescent mental health problems have a one-year period prevalence of 10-20%, depending on the population surveyed and the severity threshold[32]. The prevalence of depression rises in adolescence and major depression is found in 2-8%, particularly among females[33]. Depression is frequently associated with other psychiatric conditions[34].

Suicidal thoughts are common in adolescence. Suicide attempts are much fewer but the problem is significant. A higher number of those who attempt self harm are female, but suicide is more common in young males[35], among whom suicide rates have risen in recent years, against national trends in other age-groups (trends in the numbers of suicides are shown in Table 4.12 and Figures 4.14 and 4.15). A prior attempt and abuse of alcohol or drugs are serious risk-factors for boys, and young men in prison aged 15-24 years are six times more likely to kill themselves than their peers outside prison. The prevention of suicide is one of the key targets of the Health of the Nation[36] initiative, and presents a particular challenge in adolescent age-groups.

Eating disorders occur in under 1% of adolescents[37], and are more common in girls. Anorexia nervosa and bulimia nervosa are the main conditions and their onset peaks in adolescence[38].

Figure 4.14: *Registered deaths from suicides and undetermined injury (all ages), England, 1969-92*

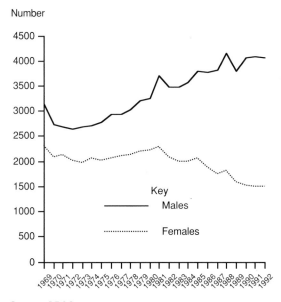

Source: OPCS

99

Table 4.12: *Registered deaths from suicide plus undetermined injury in England 1969-92*

Year	All ages		Aged 15-19 years	
	Males	Females	Males	Females
1969	3140	2303	73	36
1970	2739	2090	75	30
1971	2700	2130	65	36
1972	2647	2004	68	48
1973	2684	1976	64	43
1974	2713	2058	85	40
1975	2768	2011	98	50
1976	2945	2069	88	48
1977	2941	2094	92	47
1978	3031	2130	100	51
1979	3217	2201	118	54
1980	3262	2219	116	57
1981	3709	2279	174	67
1982	3467	2084	124	46
1983	3482	2002	128	45
1984	3561	1983	130	37
1985	3792	2052	144	49
1986	3771	1889	159	58
1987	3813	1750	170	52
1988	4150	1805	193	59
1989	3793	1590	164	58
1990	4070	1524	160	48
1991	4078	1489	166	51
1992	4052	1489	130	40

Source: OPCS

Figure 4.15: *Registered deaths from suicides and undetermined injury (ages 15-19 years), England, 1969-92*

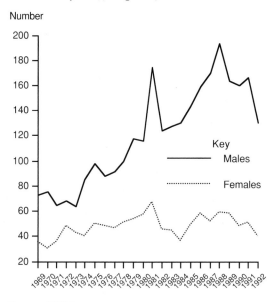

Source: OPCS

References

1. Allied Dunbar National Fitness Survey. *A report on activity patterns and fitness levels commissioned by the Sports Council and the Health Education Authority: main findings.* London: Sports Council, 1992.
2. Royal College of Physicians of London. *Smoking and the young: a report of a working party of the Royal College of Physicians.* London: Royal College of Physicians, 1992.
3. West P, Macintyre E, Annandale E, Hunt K. Social class and health in youth: findings from the West of Scotland twenty-07 study. *Soc Sci Med* 1990; **30**: 665-73.
4. West P. Inequalities? Social class differentials in British youth. *Soc Sci Med* 1988; **27**: 291.
5. Slater M. *Health for all our children: achieving appropriate healthcare for black and minority ethnic children and their families.* London: Action for Sick Children, 1993.
6. King's Fund Institute. *Purchasing for Health.* London: King's Fund Institute, 1993.
7. Hillman M. *Children, transport and the quality of life.* London: Policy Studies Institute, 1993.
8. Challener J. Health education in secondary schools - is it working? A study of 1,418 Cambridgeshire pupils. *Public Health* 1990; **104**: 195-205.
9. Department of Health. *The Diets of British Schoolchildren.* London: HMSO, 1989 (Report on Health and Social Subjects no. 36).
10. Nelson M, White J, Rhodes C. Haemoglobin, ferritin, and iron intakes in British children aged 12-14 years: a preliminary investigation. *Br J Nutr* 1993; **70**: 147-55.
11. Kanders B, Dempster DW, Lindsay R. Interaction of calcium nutrition and physical activity on bone mass in young women. *J Bone Min Res* 1988; **3**: 145-9.
12. Haas JD, Fairchild MW. Summary and conclusions of the International Conference on Iron Deficiency and Behavioural Development, October 10-12, 1988. *Am J Clin Nutr* 1989; **50**: 703-5.
13. Crawley HF. The energy, nutrient and food intakes of teenagers aged 16-17 years in Britain. *Br J Nutr* 1993; **70**: 15-26.
14. Department of Health. *Dietary Reference Values for Food Energy and Nutrients for the United Kingdom.* London: HMSO, 1991 (Report on Health and Social Subjects no. 41).
15. Charlton A. The Brigantia Smoking Survey: a general review. Public education about cancer. *UICC Tech Rep Ser* 1984; **77**: 92-102.
16. Goddard E. *Why children start smoking: an enquiry carried out by Social Survey Division of OPCS on behalf of the Department of Health.* London: HMSO, 1993
17. Health Education Authority. *Tomorrow's Young Adults: 9-15 year olds look at alcohol, drugs, exercise and smoking.* London: Health Education Authority, 1992.
18. Office of Population Censuses and Surveys. *Smoking among secondary school children in 1992: a survey carried out by the Social Services Division of OPCS on behalf of the Department of Health, the Welsh Office and the Scottish Office Home and Health Department.* London: HMSO, 1993.
19. Home Office Standing Conference on Crime Prevention. *A report of the Working Group on Young People and Alcohol.* London: Home Office, 1987.
20. Home Office. Statistics of Drug Addicts Notified to the Home Office, United Kingdom 1992. *Home Office Stat Bull* 1993; 93/15.
21. Department of Health. *Drugs and solvents: you and your child.* London: HMSO, 1993.
22. Wellings K, Field J, Johnson A, Wandsworth J, Bradshaw S. *Sexual Behaviour in Britain.* London: Penguin, (in press).
23. Rosenheim M, Testa M, eds. *Early Parenthood and Coming of Age in the 1990s.* New Brunswick: Rutgers University Press, 1992.
24. Mellanby A, Phelps F, Tripp JH. Teenagers, sex and risk taking. *BMJ* 1993 **307**: 25.
25. Royal College of Obstetricians and Gynaecologists. *Report of the RCOG Working Party on Unplanned Pregnancy.* London: Royal College of Obstetricians and Gynaecologists, 1991. Chairs: John Loundon, Sir Alexander Turnbull.
26. Nyman V. Going Dutch - a pipe dream? *Br J Family Planning* 1993; **19**: 200-3.
27. Rademakers J. *Contraception and Interaction.* Utrecht: University of Utrecht, 1991 [MD thesis].
28. Epstein R, Rice P, Wallace P. Teenagers' health concerns: implications for primary health care. *J R Coll Gen Pract* 1989; **39**: 247-9.
29. Department of Health. *Priorities and planning guidance 1994/95.* Heywood (Lancashire): Department of Health, 1993 (Executive Letter: EL(93)54).
30. Allen I. *Family planning and pregnancy counselling projects for young people.* London: Policy Studies Institute, 1992.
31. British Medical Association. *Confidentiality and People under 16: guidance issued jointly by the British Medical Association, General Medical Services Committee, Health Education Authority, Brook Advisory Centres, Family Planning Association and the Royal College of General Practitioners.* London: BMA, 1993.
32. Rutter M, Graham P, Chadwick O, Yule W. Adolescent Turmoil: fact or fiction? *J Child Psychol Psychiatry* 1976; **17**: 35-56.
33. Harrington R. *Affective disorders.* In: Rutter M, Taylor E, Hersov L, eds. *Child and Adolescent Psychiatry: modern approaches* (3rd edn). Oxford: Blackwell Scientific Publications (in press).
34. Harrington RC, Fudge H, Rutter M, Pickles A, Hill J. Adult outcomes of childhood and adolescent depression: 1. Psychiatric status. *Arch Gen Psychiatry* 1990; **47**: 465-73.
35. Hawton K, Fagg J. Deliberate self-poisoning and self-injury in adolescents. A study of characteristics and trends in Oxford, 1976-89. *Br J Psychiatry* 1992; **161**: 816-23.

101

36. Department of Health. *The Health of the Nation: a strategy for health in England.* London: Department of Health, 1992 (Cm. 1986).
37. Whitaker A, Johnson J, Shaffer D, et al. Uncommon troubles in young people. Prevalence estimates of selected psychiatric disorders in a non-referred population. *Arch Gen Psychiatry* 1990; **47**: 487-96.
38. Steinhausen HC. *Anorexia and Bulimia Norvosa.* In: Rutter M, Taylor E, Hersov L, eds. *Child and Adolescent Psychiatry: modern approaches* (3rd edn). Oxford: Blackwell Scientific Publications (in press).

(e)   Social factors

(i)   Child protection

The incidence of child abuse in England is not known precisely, but improved public awareness, better professional recognition and society's unwillingness to tolerate the abuse of young people have led to increased reporting and identification[1]. Up to half of all abusive episodes occur in adolescence[2], with sexual and psychological abuse predominating[2]. Some episodes begin during adolescence and are not simply a continuation of an earlier established pattern, but abuse occurring in adolescence is far less likely to be reported to protective services than its equivalent among younger children[2].

Table 4.13 shows the numbers of young people on child protection registers by age, sex and registration category. Figures 4.16 and 4.17 show the increase in registrations for sexual abuse in girls as they pass through adolescence.

During adolescence, all socio-economic groups are equally at risk; families with step-parents are especially vulnerable[2]. The detrimental consequences of psychological, sexual and physical maltreatment on adolescent adjustment may be severe and an association has been found with contemporaneous and later suicide attempts, drug and alcohol misuse, running away, promiscuity and delinquency[2].

(ii)   Children looked after by Local Authorities

Following implementation of the Children Act 1989[3], the term 'in care' was replaced by 'looked after'. The majority of such children are looked after in foster homes, reflecting a move away from care in childrens' homes. Figures 4.18 and 4.19 and Table 4.14 show the distribution of looked after children by age and sex.

The Children Act 1989[3] Regulations require regular assessment and examination, but comprehensive data about the physical and mental health and educational attainment of this group have not been available[4,5,6]. The 'Looking After Children' schedules, presently undergoing pilot studies, will help to provide this information[7]. The National Child Development Study showed 24% of children looked after at 16 years-of-age were receiving special education compared with 2% of those who had never been looked after[5].

102

Table 4.13: *Rates* and numbers of children and young people on child protection registers by age, sex, and registration category, England, at 31 March 1993*

	All categories	Neglect	Physical injury	Sexual abuse	Emotional abuse	Grave concern	Numbers
All ages	23	5	9	6	2	2	32500
Under 1 year	51	17	24	6	3	6	2300
1 to 4 years	27	8	12	5	3	2	9900
5 to 9 years	22	5	8	6	3	2	10000
10 to 15 years	19	3	7	7	2	1	9100
16 years and over	5	1	2	2	0	0	1100
Males							
All ages	21	5	9	4	2	2	16000
Under 1 year	50	16	24	5	3	6	1200
1 to 4 years	28	8	13	4	2	2	5100
5 to 9 years	23	5	9	5	3	2	5250
10 to 15 years	16	3	6	4	2	1	4100
16 years and over	3	0	1	2	2	1	400
Females							
All ages	24	5	8	8	2	2	16400
Under 1 year	53	7	24	7	3	6	1200
1 to 4 years	27	8	11	5	3	2	4800
5 to 9 years	22	5	7	8	3	1	4700
10 to 15 years	22	3	7	11	2	1	5000
16 years and over	6	1	2	3	1	0	700

*Rates per 10,000 population in each age and sex group; children may be registered in more than one category, so the sum of the columns may exceed the total rate for all categories.

Source: Government Statistical Service

Figure 4.16: *Rates of males on child protection register by age, sex, and category of abuse, England*

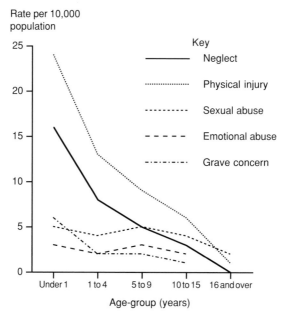

Source: Government Statistical Service

Figure 4.17: *Rates of females on child protection register by age, sex, and category of abuse, England*

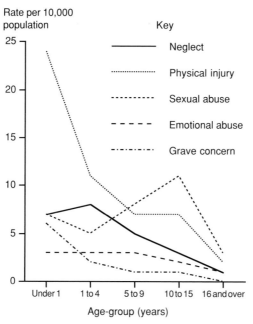

Source: Government Statistical Service

(iii)   *Divorce*

The divorce rate in England is one of the highest in Europe and, if present trends continue, one in four children will experience breakdown in their parents' marriage by the age of 16 years[8]. Young people whose families undergo disruption and change are more likely to experience social, educational and health problems than those whose families remain intact[9]. Girls who become part of a step-family by the age of 16 years run twice the risk of becoming teenage mothers and giving birth to their baby outside marriage; are at three times greater risk of leaving home before their 18th birthday because of disagreements or ill feelings; and are four times more likely to marry before the age of 20 years than those who continue to live with both parents. Boys and girls alike run twice the risk of leaving school to seek employment at the age of 16 years[10].

(iv)   *Violence*

Much of our knowledge of adolescents and violence comes from the United States of America (USA), where violence among young people is said to be reaching "epidemic" proportions[11]. The causes are multiple: social and physical environment, family, poverty, social control and individual psychological make-up all interact[12]. Most violent acts arise spontaneously from arguments between family members and between friends of the same age, race and gender[11].

Early exposure to violence and abuse, physical, emotional and sexual, as a victim or a witness, and exposure to corporal punishment, are all associated with increased rates of adolescent violence[13]. Male socialisation and peer group pressure have also been identified as contributing to a predisposition to violence[14], and there may be an association between media violence and aggression[15]. Adolescent murderers are more likely to have criminally violent families, to be gang members, to have severe educational problems and to abuse alcohol[13], and to participate in repeated viewing of violent or pornographic videos[12].

Table 4.14: *Children looked after by Local Authorities, England, at 31 March 1992*

	Males	Females	Males %	Females %
Total	28730	25620		
Under 1 year	750	660	2.6	2.6
1 to 4 years	4200	3700	14.6	14.4
5 to 9 years	6100	5300	21.2	20.7
10 to 15 years	11400	9800	39.7	38.3
16 to 17 years	6000	5900	20.9	23.0
18 years and over	280	260	1.0	1.0

Source: Government Statistical Service

Figure 4.18: *Males looked after by Local Authorities by age-group, England, at 31 March 1992*

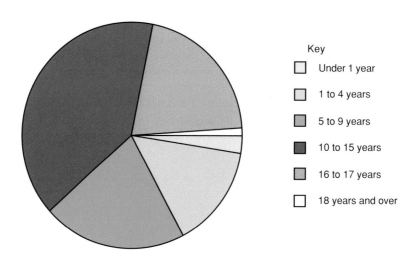

Key

☐ Under 1 year

☐ 1 to 4 years

☐ 5 to 9 years

■ 10 to 15 years

☐ 16 to 17 years

☐ 18 years and over

Source: Government Statistical Service

Figure 4.19: *Females looked after by Local Authorities by age-group, England, at 31 March 1992*

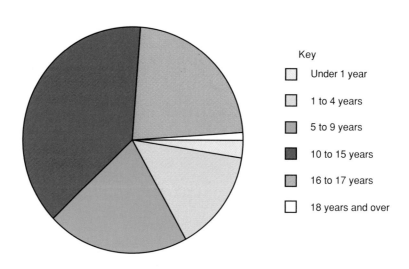

Key

☐ Under 1 year

☐ 1 to 4 years

☐ 5 to 9 years

■ 10 to 15 years

☐ 16 to 17 years

☐ 18 years and over

Source: Government Statistical Service

(v) *Unauthorised school absence*

Against a background of concern over the serious educational and social consequences associated with unauthorised absence from school of children of compulsory school age, the Department for Education (DFE) published information on rates of unauthorised absence in November 1993[16]. The national tables indicated that, in the 1992-93 school year up to and including 28 May 1993, 12% of young people in maintained secondary schools had engaged in unauthorised absence at least once. An average of 24 half-days were lost per absent pupil.

To provide practical help to schools that experience difficulty in maintaining high levels of attendance, the DFE supported substantial projects put forward by local education authorities to reduce unauthorised absence. Advice on the categorisation of pupil absence will be issued for consultation in 1994. This emphasises the importance of regular school attendance and encourages schools to investigate unauthorised absence.

(vi) *Employment*

Although adolescents are legally required to attend full-time education until the age of 16 years, young people are legally able to work 2 hours daily between 0700 and 1900 hours from the age of 13 years[17]. Whilst the numbers involved are not known, some 35-40% of children aged 11 to 15 years may have part-time jobs, and the income from this type of work may make a significant contribution to the household budget[18,19].

Adolescent unemployment has been higher than the general level of unemployment in the population over the last 20 years (see Table 4.15 and Figure 4.20). Surveys indicate that the adolescent share of the job market sometimes falls irrespective of whether the market is expanding or stagnating, and obtaining work is particularly difficult for those with less education, those who leave school early and those with little work experience. Studies show a link between employment and psychological well-being in young people[19], and that unemployment may have an adverse effect[20].

Below the age at which adolescents seek employment they may be affected by their parents' unemployment. There is conflicting evidence on the effects of parental unemployment but it is usually accompanied by difficult material circumstances, increased stress and changing roles[21,22].

(vii) *Homelessness*

There is no clear definition of homelessness. One approach is to consider a spectrum of housing needs from sleeping rough on the streets through various types of insecure and unsatisfactory accommodation (eg, hostels or bed-and-breakfast 'hotels'), to secure housing which nevertheless fails to satisfy an individual's needs[23].

Estimating the numbers of homeless adolescents is difficult. Results from the 1991 Census indicate that 2,439 people under 18 years-of-age in England were sleeping rough, or in common lodging houses or hostels. This is only an estimate as the data did not take account of those in bed-and-breakfast accommodation. Researchers have noted increasing youth homelessness[24,25].

The combination of factors resulting in homelessness is complex. Explanations include difficulties faced by unskilled young people in the labour market and attempting to escape an abusing family or inadequate child care placement[26,27]. Adolescents may be homeless in their own right or, especially when younger, as part of a homeless family.

The difficulties in developing policies for homeless adolescents are compounded by the paucity of information about the size and nature of the problem and the wide range of professionals and organisations involved.

Little is known about the extent of prostitution among the homeless population in England, although the problem is sometimes alluded to[28] and may be a more feasible option for young people[29], with the concomitant risks of sexually transmitted diseases, including HIV/AIDS, and injury from violence.

Figure 4.20: *Percentage unemployed by age-group and sex, United Kingdom, 1974-89*

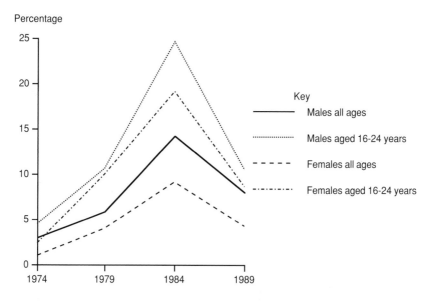

Source: Labour Force Statistics OECD

Table 4.15: *Percentage unemployment by age-group and sex, United Kingdom, 1974-89*

	1974		1979		1984		1989	
	M	F	M	F	M	F	M	F
All ages	3.0	0.9	5.8	3.9	14.2	9.1	8.0	4.2
Aged 16 to 24 years	4.4	2.3	10.6	10.0	24.6	19.1	10.5	8.6

M = Male, F = Female
Source: Labour Force Statistics, OECD

References

1. Meadow R, ed. *ABC of child abuse.* London: British Medical Journal, 1993.
2. Rutter M, Taylor E, Hersov L, eds. *Child and Adolescent Psychiatry: modern approaches* (3rd edn). Oxford: Blackwell Scientific Publications (in press).
3. *The Children Act 1989.* London: HMSO, 1989.
4. Kahan B, ed. *Child care research, policy and practice.* London: Hodder and Stoughton, 1989.
5. Bamford F. *The physical health of children in care: research needs.* In: Bamford F, Wolkind SN. *The physical and mental health of children in care.* Swindon: Economic and Social Research Council, 1988.
6. Wolkind SN. *The mental health of children in care: research needs.* In: Bamford F, Wolkind SN. *The physical and mental health of children in care.* Swindon: Economic and Social Research Council, 1988.
7. Parker R, Ward H, Jackson S, Aldgate J, Wedge P. *Looking after children. Assessing Outcomes in Child Care: the report of an independent working party established by the Department of Health.* London: HMSO, 1991.
8. Haskey J. Children in families broken by divorce. *Pop Trends* 1990; **61**: 34-42.
9. Joseph Rowntree Foundation. *Children living in reordered families.* York: Joseph Rowntree Foundation (in press).
10. Kiernan KE. The impact of family disruption in childhood on transitions made in young adult life. *Pop Trends* 1992; **46**: 213-34.
11. Prothrow-Stith, D. The epidemic of violence and its impact on the health care system. *Henry Ford Hospital Med J* 1990; **38**: 175-7.
12. Bailey S. Fast forward to violence: violent visual imaging and serious juvenile crime. *Criminal Justice Matters* 1993; **11**: 6-7.
13. Sege RD. Adolescent Violence. *Curr Opinion Paediatr* 1992; **4**: 575-81.
14. Russell DEH. Pornography and rape: a causal model. *Political Psychol* 1988; **9**: 41-73.
15. Heath L, Bresolin LB, Rinaldi RC. Effects of media violence on children: a review of the literature. *Arch Gen Psychiatry* 1989; **46**: 376-9.
16. Department for Education and Science. *National unauthorised absence tables 1992-93.* London: Department for Education and Science, 1993.
17. *Health and Safety at Work Act 1974.* London: HMSO, 1974.
18. Avery JG, Jackson HR. *Children and their accidents.* London: Edward Arnold, 1993.
19. Fyfe A. *Child Labour.* Cambridge: Policy Press, 1989.
20. Winefield AH, Tiggemann M, Winefield HR. The psychological impact of unemployment and unsatisfactory employment in young men and women: longitudinal and cross-sectional data. *Br J Psychol* 1991; **82**: 473-86.
21. Stavia B, Svensson PG. *Vulnerability in the labour market: unemployment in Europe in health policy development for disadvantaged groups.* Oslo: Scandinavian University Press, 1992.
22. Wilson SH, Waller GM. Unemployment and health: a review. *Public Health* 1993; **107**: 153-62.
23. Faculty of Public Health Medicine, Royal College of Physicians of London. *Homelessness and health.* London: Royal College of Physicians (in press).
24. Bramley G, Doozen K, Leather P, Murie A, Watson E, eds. *Homelessness and the London housing market.* Bristol: School for Advanced Urban Studies, 1988.
25. Shelter. *Building for the future: Shelter's 25th anniversary report.* London: Shelter, 1991.
26. White A. *Health in the inner city.* London: Heinemann, 1989.
27. Anderson I, Kemp P, Quilgars D. *Single Homeless People: a report for the Department of the Environment.* London: HMSO, 1993.
28. Marshall EJ, Reed JL. Psychiatric morbidity in homeless women. *Br J Psychiatry* 1992; vol: RP.
29. Fisher K, Collins J, eds. *Homelessness, health care and welfare provision.* London: Routledge, 1993.

(f)   Health services for adolescents

The provision of health services for adolescents is influenced by a lack of recognition that adolescents have particular and definable needs. This is most marked in secondary care where there is a clear professional and institutional demarcation between child and adult services and where no single specialty has a remit for the care of adolescents equivalent to the role of paediatricians and geriatricians in the care of young children and old people. This has the greatest impact on young people with disabilities or chronic and life-threatening conditions where medical science has secured their survival beyond childhood into young adulthood. The need is to identify a clinician to take responsibility for these patients during adolescence to provide the expertise and continuity of care required by young people and their families.

Reasons for admitting patients to paediatric or adult facilities may be arbitrary and depend, for example, on the availability of facilities rather than the degree of maturity of the patient. Admission to an adult general surgical, urological, or orthopaedic ward may be particularly inappropriate for adolescents given the range of degenerative and malignant conditions that may be treated on such wards. Long periods of stay - for example, for fractured femur, when the patient is fully alert and feels well, but is immobile - can be particularly difficult.

Only a small number of mentally disturbed adolescents need access to specialist mental health services, and many will receive help and advice from primary health care teams, school staff, social services and voluntary agencies, with the help of outreach programmes from specialist adolescent mental health services. Those with more severe psychiatric disorders may require inpatient treatment. 'Difficult to place' adolescents have challenged agencies for decades. These multiply damaged young people feel very troubled and are often difficult to care for, with extreme disorders of behaviour and emotions that often appear resistant to conventional therapeutic interventions. Although mental illness may rarely cause such problems, social and educational difficulties are often the main challenges. No single institution is sufficient and health, social services, education, voluntary and private sectors, and the criminal justice system all need to contribute in a co-ordinated way.

It has been demonstrated that general practice is an appropriate setting for adolescents to raise health concerns and receive advice on healthy lifestyles and that GPs can perform effectively in adolescent health care[1]. Adolescents see GPs more than any other health professionals[2], and further development of adolescent health services might be most effectively rooted in primary care. Work from North America has shown that the development of the specialty of adolescent medicine has augmented primary care efforts - for example, the development of services for teenage prostitutes and substance misusers, and clinics in schools and settings where homeless teenagers congregate[3]. In England, 'drop in' centres are being set up where young people can receive health care and advice.

The School Health Service (SHS) has an important part to play in the provision of health services to adolescents of school age and in providing support to help teachers to give effective health education. Teachers have professional responsibility for teaching health education, which the SHS supports by providing professional expertise for the planning and execution of the work. There has been little evaluation of the majority of school health education programmes but a study of 1,418 14-year-old secondary school pupils reporting in 1990 showed that 90% of girls and 70% of boys would like more information on health education to be included in the school curriculum[4].

References

1. Epstein R, Rice P, Wallace P. Teenagers' Health Concern: implications for primary health care professionals. *J R Coll Gen Pract* 1989; **39**: 247-9.
2. Strasburger VC, Brown RT. *Adolescent Medicine: a practical guide.* Boston: Little, Brown, 1991.
3. Malus M. Towards a separate adolescent medicine. *BMJ* 1992; **305**: 789-90.
4. Challener J. Health Education in Secondary Schools - is it working? A study of 1,418 Cambridgeshire pupils.. *Publ Health* 1990; **104**: 195-205.

(g)   Improving the health of adolescents

In adolescence, mortality and morbidity are dominated by factors and conditions reflecting adolescent risk-taking behaviour and disregard for the consequences of an unhealthy lifestyle. By contrast to the inexorable disease processes of older age-groups, however, many of the determinants of adolescent health are behavioural and lifestyle-related and ought to be amenable to intervention. Indeed, most adolescents seem to recognise that health is largely self-determined and a matter of personal responsibility[1].

Many interventions have been successful. Health professionals can help to reduce physical inactivity in adolescents[2], and promote their health in general. Head injuries from road accidents involving teenagers can be reduced by cycle helmets[3], and by understanding of the behaviours that lead to accidents[4]. The risk-factors for suicide in adolescence are complex but may include substance misuse[5], which can be prevented[6]. Unwanted pregnancies in young girls may be reduced by sex education, though knowledge by itself may be insufficient[7].

Adolescence is a stage when health-related behavioural and lifestyle patterns are established, but which may not demonstrate their health consequences until later life. Interventions in adolescence to modify health-related behaviours may therefore have major importance for individuals' long-term health and on later use of health service resources.

To be effective, adolescent health care must focus on the particular characteristics of adolescents and reflect their need for increasing autonomy and independence. The necessary development of autonomy and personal decision-making during adolescence runs counter to the acceptance of advice from others, and the views of young people must be taken into account when determining the development of appropriate health services and effective delivery of adolescent health care. Health messages for adolescents must be tailored to their needs, suitable in style and content, and designed for maximum impact, whilst remaining sensitive to race, culture and gender.

Research has identified the key role played by parents in promoting the health of young people[8] and as a source of health information[1]. Young people not only turn to parents for health advice but also use them as role models[8]. It is important, therefore, to involve parents in promoting the health of adolescents. However, parental involvement and the adolescent's need for privacy in health care must be carefully balanced as a concern for many adolescents is whether information shared in private will remain confidential[9]. Parents need to understand and to be reassured that the desire for confidentiality is a normal part of adolescent development.

Although adolescents use health services as frequently as older age-groups and for a broadly similar range of disorders, they have unique needs and represent a unique opportunity for change. Improvement of adolescent health will demand skill, understanding and patience but should be cost-effective in both the short and the long term; if prevention is indeed better than cure, a focus on adolescent health should yield great dividends.

References

1. Macfarlane A, McPherson A, McPherson K, Ahmed L. Teenagers and their health. *Arch Dis Childh* 1987; **62**: 1125-9.
2. Armstrong N. Promoting physical activity in schools. *Health Visitor* 1993; **66**: 362-4.
3. Thomas S, Acton C, Nixon J, Battistutta D, Pitt WR, Clark R. Effectiveness of bicycle helmets in preventing head injury in children: case-control study. *BMJ* (in press).
4. Farrow JA, Brissing P. Risk for DWI: a new look at gender differences in drinking and driving influences, experiences, and attitudes among new adolescent drivers. *Health Educ Q* 1990; **17** : 213-21.
5. Hawton K, Fagg J, Platt S, Hawkins M. Factors associated with suicide after parasuicide in young people. *BMJ* 1993; **306**: 1641-4.
6. Swadi H. Alcohol abuse in adolescence; an update. *Arch Dis Childh* 1993; **68**: 341-3.
7. Henderson J, Goldacre M, Yeates D. Use of hospital inpatient care in adolescence. *Arch Dis Childh* 1993; **69**; 559-63.
8. Brennan J, Oakley A, Storey P. *Young people, health and family life.* Buckingham: Open University Press (in press).
9. Council on Scientific Affairs. Confidential health services for adolescents. *JAMA* 1993; **269**: 1420-4.

CHAPTER 5

HEALTH CARE

(a)   Needs, effectiveness and outcomes

(i)   Health needs assessment

The assessment of local health care needs is a basic activity which underpins the purchasing of appropriate health care by District Health Authorities (DHAs). The Department of Health (DH) has supported these local actions by publishing epidemiologically based needs reviews, as detailed in last year's Report[1]. During 1993, this series was extended to include reviews on colorectal cancer[2], lower respiratory tract disease[3], child health services[4], family planning services[5], and drug misuse[6]. These reviews are distributed to DHAs, Family Health Services Authorities (FHSAs), Regional Health Authorities (RHAs) and universities. An evaluation of the distribution of provisional reviews found that over 90% of recipients found them useful, particularly for needs assessments, negotiations with providers and the preparation of purchasing plans or contracts. A high proportion of respondents suggested that the availability of these central reviews reduced the need for local reviews of individual services. More topics will be covered during 1994.

Health needs assessment is still in its infancy. DH has set up a project to assess local activity and progress in purchasing initiatives and to identify how this needs assessment influences local purchasing of health care.

(ii)   Basic sources of information

The health survey programme

The 1991 Health Survey for England was published in July[7], and results of the 1992 survey should be published early in 1994. The 1993 Health Survey ran throughout the year and included approximately 17,000 adults. Like the previous two surveys, and the forthcoming 1994 survey, it focused on risk factors for coronary heart disease (CHD) and stroke. From 1995, the main emphasis of the survey is likely to shift from cardiovascular disease to other topics, and children may also be included; however, key assessments in earlier surveys will be retained.

In June, the National Diet and Nutrition Survey Programme, sponsored jointly with the Ministry of Agriculture, Fisheries and Food (MAFF), concluded its fieldwork on a representative sample of British children aged 1.5-4.5 years. Plans were prepared for a survey of the diet of people aged 65 years or over, and fieldwork should begin in late 1994. A survey of Asian infant feeding practices is also planned.

The National Psychiatric Morbidity Survey started during 1993 and should be completed in 1994; a series of reports will follow.

Morbidity statistics from general practice

The 4th National Study of Morbidity Statistics from General Practice collected morbidity data for each consultation in 60 general practices and 500,000 patients for the year to the end of August 1992. Data preparation and analysis continued during 1993 and preliminary results and a full report should be published during 1994.

Public Health Information Strategy

In 1990, DH set up the Public Health Information Strategy (PHIS) programme to ensure that it collects the information required to support its objectives in the most cost-effective way. The final strategy report was completed in September 1992. During 1993, the strategy team concentrated on individual projects, including some related to the Health of the Nation key areas of mental health and accidents. Work on accident prevention was endorsed by the Inter-Departmental Accidents Prevention Task Force and will be taken forward during 1994. A project on mothers' and babies' health is also in progress.

As a result of PHIS, a strategic forward programme of health surveys is being co-ordinated within the Department. The overall information strategy is being reviewed to ensure that its aims and objectives are still relevant.

Information management and technology

The National Health Service (NHS) Management Executive's Information Management and Technology Strategy for the NHS in England was launched in December 1992[8]. Good progress continues with key projects to share information across the NHS, including the development of an NHS-wide networking capability, the replacement of NHS numbers with a common single identifier and the provision of strict protocols to ensure confidentiality and security of data. Further guidance on a central approval process for information management and technology investments of or above £1 million has been developed. The National Casemix Office is completing the revision of Health Resource Groups information to be used to price contracts for acute inpatients, and to provide better comparative information. Work continues on cost assessments in other health care sectors to help purchasers understand and plan for the health care needs of their local populations.

Clinical terms project

A two-year project to develop a thesaurus of coded, nationally agreed clinical terms and groupings, expanding on the Read codes used in primary care[9], was set up by the NHS Management Executive and medical and other health care professions in April 1992[10]. Forty-three working groups have identified terms to ensure that clinical information - including signs, symptoms, diagnoses and prescribed medications - can be translated and understood on computers across the NHS. The medical component of the thesaurus should be released by mid-1994, with terms for allied professions and nurses becoming available in late-1994 and mid-1995, respectively.

(iii) National confidential enquiries

The Report for 1992[11] described the purpose of confidential enquiry, the avenues of investigation that are followed and the method by which such enquiries are conducted. It emphasised the need to maintain confidentiality and to use procedures that allow no feedback on individual cases to patients or their relatives.

During 1993, good progress was made on all five national confidential enquiries. The reports of the Confidential Enquiries into Peri-operative Deaths (see page 123) and into Stillbirths and Deaths in Infancy (see page 134) were published, and the report of the Confidential Enquiries into Maternal Deaths was prepared for publication early in 1994 (see page 131). Reports of the Enquiries into Counselling for Genetic Disorders and into Homicides and Suicides by Mentally Ill People are expected to be published during 1994 and 1995, respectively.

It is important that the recommendations of confidential enquiries for improvements in training, clinical practice and service provision are implemented to improve the quality and outcome of care in their respective fields.

(iv) Quality of service and effectiveness of care

As outlined in last year's Report[12], the identification of benefits in terms of improved health, patient satisfaction and improved quality of life - or clinical outcome - is a key component in demonstrating the quality of clinical care. During 1993, the Clinical Outcomes Group (COG) continued its work and set up sub-groups for primary care, to draw up proposals for audit in primary care and to assess the interface with audit in secondary care, and for patients. COG will also consider aspects of the development of clinical guidelines as a tool to improve clinical effectiveness. The change in emphasis from uniprofessional to multiprofessional audit was encouraged by the publication of *Clinical Audit: meeting and improving standards in healthcare*[13] in July 1993, and a report on the evolution of clinical audit was prepared for publication early in 1994. A working party was set up to consider the need for advice on future funding arrangements when responsibility for audit is devolved to purchasers, and its report should also be published early in 1994.

During 1993, DH allocated £50.1 million to support audit in hospital and community health services, and £12.2 million for audit in primary care. The principal objective of these programmes is to ensure that clinical audit becomes firmly embedded in the clinical practice of all health care professionals.

(v) *Clinical standards and guidelines*

DHAs and general practitioner (GP) fundholders continue to develop more sophisticated approaches to purchasing health care on the basis of information about the effectiveness of clinical interventions. DH continued to support the publication of Effective Health Care bulletins; during 1993 these covered the treatment of depression in primary care[14], cholesterol screening and treatment[15], and brief interventions to reduce harm from alcohol misuse[16]. Various methods of using research-based information to influence purchasing decisions have been explored as part of the NHS research and development strategy. For instance, the Getting Research into Practice (GRIP) programme was assessing the use of evidence on the treatment of pre-term labour, dysmenorrhoea, stroke and glue ear to inform purchasing discussions and to improve the efficacy and cost-effectiveness of health care.

The development of clinical standards and guidelines has a long history, but their value has been highlighted by the need to establish standards for clinical audit. Clinical guidelines need to take account of research evidence and be widely acceptable to health care professionals. The NHS Management Executive therefore started a development programme for the use of high-quality clinical guidelines in the purchasing of health care. DHAs and GP fundholders were asked to select at least one clinical guideline related to radiology, asthma, diabetes mellitus, heart disease, leg ulcers, neonatal respiratory distress syndrome, and head injury in the development of purchasing contracts for 1994/95[17]. These seven topics were chosen on the basis of existing clinical guidelines that had been developed and endorsed by the relevant professional bodies; were based on research evidence of clinical effectiveness; were practical and affordable and, where appropriate, multidisciplinary; and took account of patient choices and values. However, such clinical guidelines are not intended to prescribe detailed management for individual patients.

(vi) *Clinical audit in primary care*

Continuing medical education for GPs continues to be supported by the Postgraduate Education Allowance (PGEA) programme, but there is also a need to encourage multidisciplinary professional development for primary health care. Some primary health care teams have identified educational requirements and the steps required to meet these, including portfolio learning for individuals. A wide range of courses is now available on practice management, multidisciplinary teamwork, information technology and clinical topics.

Clinical multidisciplinary audit should be an integral part of continuing professional development, and its educational value is being increasingly recognised. However, the links between audit and educational programmes still need to be strengthened. Multidisciplinary audit of primary care can also improve teamwork and encourage all members of primary health care teams to set standards and evaluate these within practices, between practices and between primary and secondary care.

(vii)   Health outcomes

Central initiatives to take forward the assessment of health outcomes of care, including the establishment of the Central Health Outcomes Unit (CHOU) and the UK Clearing House on Outcomes, the development of health outcome indicators and the setting up of an outcomes research and development programme, have been described in previous Reports[18,19] and continue to evolve. The definition of health outcomes, published in the 1991 Report[18], was revised to an "Attributable effect of intervention or its lack on a previous health state".

Population health outcome models and indicators

Following a report of the Chief Medical Officer's Working Group on Outcome Indicators the CHOU commissioned the Faculty of Public Health Medicine of the Royal College of Physicians of London to undertake a feasibility study of potential indicators, and subsequently commissioned the University of Surrey to analyse the indicators recommended in the Faculty's report[20]. These indicators were health outcome indicators for health problems or conditions where the NHS had an important role. In September, DH published a consultation document *Population Health Outcome Indicators for the NHS*[21], alongside the Faculty's report[20] on the feasibility study. The consultation document included a summary of the Working Group report; descriptions of 40 indicators that covered maternal and child health, general health and mental health, with specifications of health objectives, data requirements, sources of information and guidance on data interpretation; and data tables, maps and scatter-plots based on analysis of data at national, regional and local level as appropriate for each of the 40 indicators, including confidence limits wherever possible.

For example, there is a substantial variation in mortality from peptic ulcer between NHS Regions and Districts which needs further explanation. Mortality from peptic ulcer is the extreme clinical end-point of a sequence of events including individual susceptibility, environmental and lifestyle factors, local and regional incidence and prevalence, and the risk and treatment of complications such as haemorrhage or perforation; several health interventions may influence this sequence at different stages. Figure 5.1 is an illustrative population health outcome model which shows how these factors may interact in the population. Such models should provide a framework to support more systematic investigations of poor local outcome values.

The consultation exercise, which was completed in December, has been very positive. Constructive comments were made on the details of individual indicators, but most respondents welcomed the initiative and broadly agreed with the approach and methods used. However, dependence on current routine data means that published indicators were not always those most useful to health

Figure 5.1: *Factors affecting outcome of peptic ulcer*

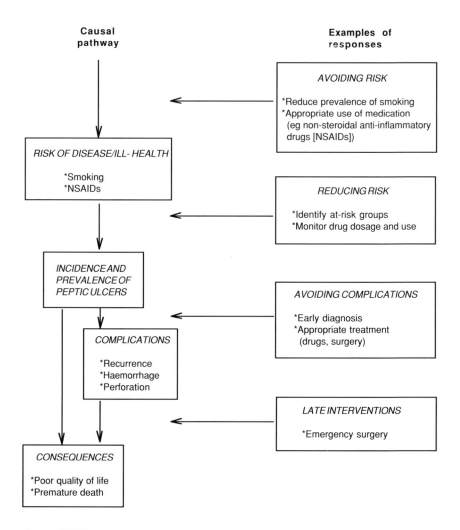

Source: CHOU

services, and CHOU will set up multidisciplinary Working Groups to specify population health outcome models, new health outcome indicators and requirements for new data collection on each of 10 health topics over two years starting in April 1994.

References

1. Department of Health. *On the State of the Public Health: the annual report of the Chief Medical Officer of the Department of Health for the year 1992.* London: HMSO, 1993; 107-9.

2. Mountney L, Sanderson H, Harris J. *Colorectal Cancer*. London: Department of Health, 1993 (Epidemiologically based needs assessment; report 15).
3. Anderson H, Esmail A, Hollowell J, Littlejohns P, Strachan D. *Lower Respiratory Disease*. London: Department of Health, 1993 (Epidemiologically based needs assessment; report 16).
4. Hall D. *Community Child Health Services*. London: Department of Health, 1993 (Epidemiologically based needs assessment; report 17).
5. Ashton J, Marchbank A, Mauvle P, et al. *Family Planning, Abortion and Fertility Services*. London: Department of Health, 1993 (Epidemiologically based needs assessment; report 18).
6. Strang J. *Drug Abuse*. London: Department of Health, 1993 (Epidemiologically based needs assessment; report 19).
7. Office of Population Censuses and Surveys. *Health Survey for England 1991*. London: HMSO, 1993.
8. Department of Health. *An Information Management and Technology Strategy for the NHS in England: IM&T strategy overview*. Cambridge: Information Management Group of the NHS Management Executive, 1992.
9. Chisholm J. The Read clinical classification. *BMJ* 1990; **300**: 1092.
10. Buckland R. The language of health. *BMJ* 1993; **306**: 287-8.
11. Department of Health. *On the State of the Public Health: the annual report of the Chief Medical Officer of the Department of Health for the year 1992*. London: HMSO, 1993; 109-10.
12. Department of Health. *On the State of the Public Health: the annual report of the Chief Medical Officer of the Department of Health for the year 1992*. London: HMSO, 1993; 110.
13. Department of Health. *Clinical audit: meeting and improving standards in healthcare*. Heywood (Lancashire): Department of Health, 1993.
14. Freemantle N, Long A, Mason J, et al. The Treatment of Depression in Primary Care. *Effective Health Care* 1993; **5**: 1-12.
15. Freemantle N, Long A, Mason J, Sheldon T, Song F, Wison C. Cholesterol: screening and treatment: what is the role of cholesterol screening and cholesterol lowering treatment? *Effective Health Care* 1993; **6**: 1-8.
16. Freemantle N, Gill P, Godfrey C, et al. Brief Interventions and Alcohol Use. *Effective Health Care* 1993; **7**: 1-14.
17. NHS Management Executive. *Improving Clinical Effectiveness*. Heywood (Lancashire): Department of Health, 1993 (Executive Letter: EL(93)115).
18. Department of Health. *On the State of the Public Health: the annual report of the Chief Medical Officer of the Department of Health for the year 1991*. London: HMSO, 1992; 81.
19. Department of Health. *On the State of the Public Health: the annual report of the Chief Medical Officer of the Department of Health for the year 1992*. London: HMSO, 1993; 110-2.
20. McColl AJ, Gulliford MC. *Population Health Outcome Indicators for the NHS: a feasibility study*. London: Faculty of Public Health Medicine of the Royal College of Physicians, 1993.
21. Department of Health. *Population Health Outcome Indicators for the NHS, 1993: England: a consultation document*. London: Department of Health, 1993.

(b)   Primary health care

(i)   *Organisation of primary care*

April 1993 saw the implementation of *Caring for People*[1]. Monitoring of the effects of this initiative indicates that the basic structural arrangements for the provision of community services are in place almost everywhere, with continued progress towards joint planning and collaborative arrangements between health and local authorities, but there remains a need to inform GPs and their colleagues in primary care about the range of services available.

Multidisciplinary teams with an appropriate mix of professional skills are essential for the provision of high-quality and cost-effective primary care. The full potential of this team approach will only be realised by effective administrative support and continued professional commitment. Local multidisciplinary training could prove to be an important part of this process; the publication of *New Worlds, New Opportunities*[2] supported the team concept and recommended that community nursing services should focus on practice populations wherever possible and practicable. Practice nurses are now firmly established in GP surgeries and undertake a wide range of tasks including general health promotion, chronic disease management, family planning and various health checks.

New arrangements for the funding of health promotion in general practice were introduced in July. Over 90% of GPs were approved to run programmes in the highest of three bands to promote health in relation to coronary heart disease (CHD) and stroke (see page 61). In addition, nearly 90% of GPs receive payments for the management of diabetes mellitus and asthma under the Chronic Disease Management Programme.

The achievement of targets under the GP contract continued to improve. By October 1993, 89% of GPs met the higher target of 90% for childhood immunisations, and 87% met the higher target for cervical cancer screening. The introduction of vaccination against *Haemophilus influenzae* type b (Hib) saw the immunisation of 90% of targeted children by 1993.

There is some evidence of increased demand for GP services outside normal surgery hours: night visit claims rose from 1.54 million in 1990/91 to 1.65 million in 1992/93. Co-operative rotas to provide out-of-hours care have become increasingly popular.

By 1 April 1993, a quarter of the population was cared for by GP fundholding practices. In April the scope of the GP fundholding scheme was expanded to include health visiting and district nursing services, dietetic and chiropody services, mental health outpatient and community services, and health services for people with learning disabilities. The aim is to extend the benefits achieved by GP fundholders to patients who need support in the community. GP fundholders are particularly well placed to determine the services wanted by patients and the way in which existing services are provided, and are increasingly involved with hospital clinicians and managers in discussions about the local development of agreed guidelines for care.

(ii)   *Prescribing*

NHS expenditure on drugs, dressings and appliances continues to increase more rapidly than for other areas of health care. In 1992/93, the primary care drugs bill increased by 13.9% (or 9.6% after allowance for inflation) compared with the previous year; this sum (of over £2.6 billion) represented 9% of total NHS expenditure, with hospital prescribing making up a further 2.2%. Increases among fundholding practices were 4% less than for non-fundholders.

Part of this increase can be accounted for by increased identification and treatment of hypertension and increased use of prophylactic treatment for asthma. Nevertheless, although most GPs prescribe more rationally and economically than their counterparts in many other developed countries, some prescribing is unnecessary, ineffective or over-expensive. The hallmarks of good prescribing practice are efficacy, safety, a lack of side-effects, and economy. To help to achieve these objectives all GPs are provided with the *British National Formulary* (BNF), the *Medicines Resource Centre (MeReC) Bulletin*, the *Drug and Therapeutics Bulletin* and *Prescribers' Journal*. Support and advice on prescribing, including the development of practice formularies, is also available from FHSA prescribing advisers - now increased to the equivalent of 180 whole-time posts.

(iii)   Professional development and clinical audit

Continuing medical education for GPs is still supported by the PGEA programme, but the need to encourage multidisciplinary professional development in primary health care is increasingly recognised. Educational requirements have been identified locally and a wide range of courses is now available on various clinical topics, practice management, multidisciplinary teamwork, and information technology.

Multidisciplinary clinical audit should be an integral part of continued professional development and the educational value of audit, and the need for stronger links between audit and educational programmes is being increasingly recognised. Methods for multidisciplinary clinical audit enable all members of primary health care teams to set standards and to evaluate their performance against these standards within practices, between practices and between primary and secondary care.

(iv)   The way ahead

Over the next few years a particular challenge for GPs and other members of primary care teams will be the need to deliver an increasing range of services in a community setting whilst still meeting the demand from patients for basic primary care consultations. The ability of primary care teams to respond and to adapt to these changing needs and pressures in recent years has accelerated this process of change. The next few years are likely to see even greater diversity in the services provided by GPs and their professional colleagues in primary care.

Many GPs will acquire additional specialist skills and the career path in general practice is likely to broaden to reflect changes in the NHS and in society at large. Increased ability to assess the needs of their practice populations, and knowledge about clinical audit, the effectiveness of clinical interventions, resource allocation, and general aspects of public health will accompany GPs' increasing participation in the purchasing and guidance of secondary care services.

References

1.   Department of Health. *Caring for People*. London: Department of Health, 1993.
2.   Department of Health. *New Worlds, New Opportunities: nursing in primary health care*. Heywood (Lancashire): Department of Health, 1993.

(c)   Hospital services

(i)   *Specialised services*

As the NHS reforms continue to be implemented, anxieties have been expressed about the ability of the contracting system to respond to the needs of patients who require certain specialised services. This issue was investigated by the Clinical Standards Advisory Group (CSAG), who looked in particular at services for neonatal intensive care, cystic fibrosis, childhood leukaemia and coronary artery bypass surgery and angioplasty[1]. Although variations in provision around the country were identified, no evidence was found that this was attributable to the NHS reforms.

The concerns expressed by the CSAG about the needs for appropriate purchasing and contracting arrangements for specialised services were addressed in the Government's response[2] to the report. The NHS Management Executive introduced streamlined arrangements for purchasing of tertiary extra-contractual referrals in February[3], and issued advice on contracting for specialised services in November[4].

(ii)   *Cancer*

Cancer is the second most common cause of death after CHD: about one in three people will develop cancer at some time of their life, and one in four people will die of the disease. The total numbers of cancers registered in England and Wales rose by over 20% between 1979 and 1988. In part, this increase reflects improved ascertainment and an increasing number of elderly people, but there are some indications of a rise in age-standardised cancer incidence, although the reasons are not fully understood. Survival rates for cancer have improved only modestly in the past 20 years. Early diagnosis either by screening or prompt detection and referral of symptomatic disease remain key elements of policies to improve both the quality and length of life, and are supported by the inclusion of cancers as a key area in the strategy for health (see page 63)[5].

Outcome may be improved if patients are treated in or under the direction of centres which have certain minimum levels of clinical activity and where individual clinicians can gain and maintain experience, and multidisciplinary clinical teams can be established. The benefits of such special expertise have been most clearly established for the rarer cancers.

During 1993, the Chief Medical Officers of England and Wales established an Expert Advisory Group on cancer; its first task will be to provide a policy framework for the commissioning of high-quality cancer services. In June, a group chaired by Dr Christopher Paine, President of the Royal College of Radiologists, provided a report on specialist cancer services in London as part of a wider review of the capital's health services (see page 187). This report noted the existence of 15 cancer centres in London and proposed that this number should be reduced to eight larger centres, and identified a need for improved general oncology services in District General Hospitals (DGHs).

(iii)   National Confidential Enquiry into Peri-operative Deaths

The National Confidential Enquiry into Peri-operative Deaths (NCEPOD) issued its report covering the year 1991/92, in September 1993[6]. The report analyses specific operative procedures over all surgical specialties and notes an increased response rate from surgeons and anaesthetists, although this is still only about 70%. Standards are shown to be generally excellent, but some deficits in care are highlighted. Causes for concern include examples of inappropriate surgery in patients known to be dying, inadequate pre-operative preparation, the occurrence of fatal pulmonary emboli, inappropriate use of intravenous fluids, inadequate anaesthetic monitoring and instances of surgeons operating outside their area of expertise.

The report comments on resource and management issues, including the availability of intensive care and other post-operative facilities, the supervision of trainees, the need for dedicated emergency operating theatres, the use of locum staff and the low frequency of post-mortem examinations to confirm the causes of death.

A series of recommendations identify where responsibility lies to tackle problems described in the report. Despite improvements, some of these problems have also been described in previous reports, and DH is supporting work to explore how NCEPOD's findings can be utilised more effectively, including a proposed conference to be hosted by the Royal College of Surgeons of England to review the evidence on thromboprophylaxis, which will be chaired by the Chief Medical Officer.

References

1. Clinical Standards Advisory Group. *Access to and Availability of Specialist Services: report of a CSAG Committee.* London: HMSO, 1993.
2. Department of Health. *Government response to the reports by the Clinical Standards Advisory Group on Access to and Availability of Specialist Services.* Heywood (Lancashire): Department of Health, 1993.
3. Department of Health. *Guidance on operation of notification arrangements for tertiary extra-contractual referrals.* Heywood (Lancashire): Department of Health, 1993 (Health Service Guidelines: HSG(93)8).
4. Department of Health. *Contracting for specialised services.* Heywood (Lancashire): Department of Health, 1993 (Executive Letter: EL(93)98).
5. Department of Health. *The Health of the Nation: a strategy for health in England.* London: HMSO, 1992 (Cm. 1986).
6. Campling GA, Devlin HB, Hoile RW, et al. *The Report of the National Confidential Enquiry into Peri-operative Deaths: 1991/92.* London: National Confidential Enquiry into Peri-operative Deaths, 1993.

(d)   Diabetes mellitus

The 1989 St Vincent meeting on diabetes care and research brought together representatives from Government health departments, health professionals and patients with diabetes mellitus from 32 European countries. The aim of the meeting was to make recommendations to improve the quality of life and life expectancy of people with diabetes mellitus; its conclusions and recommendations were summarised in the St Vincent Declaration[1].

In July 1992, Ministers announced the setting up of a Joint DH/British Diabetic Association Task Force, chaired by Professor David Shaw, to advise on the implementation of the recommendations in England and their relative priority. The Task Force proposed a work programme which included the setting up of subgroups to advise it on the implementation of any recommendations.

Reference

1. Diabetes Mellitus in Europe: a problem at all ages in all countries: a model for prevention and self care: a meeting organised by WHO and IDF Europe: proceedings. *Giornale Italiano di Diabetologia* 1990; **10** (**suppl**).

(e)   Asthma

The prevalence of asthma sufficiently severe to require regular medical supervision is 4-6% in children and about 4% in adults[1]. The prevalence of wheezing in children over a 12-month period may be as high as 12-15%[1]. Hospital admissions for asthma have increased and finished consultant episodes with a diagnosis of asthma now account for some 4.5% of all episodes with a diagnosis among children under 15 years-of-age. The number of GP prescriptions for asthma increased from 14.87 million in 1982 to 29.26 million in 1992. Although there has been a fall in deaths from asthma under the age of 65 years, total deaths from asthma have only fallen slightly to 1,655 in England in 1992.

The reasons for the apparently increased prevalence of asthma and other atopic conditions are not known, but an increase has also been observed in other countries such as New Zealand[2] and Sweden[3]. One factor may be increased recognition and a shift in diagnostic patterns, particularly among children who might once have been thought to have 'wheezy bronchitis'. Environmental tobacco smoke and increased maternal smoking may also affect childhood asthma[4]. There has also been public concern about the possible effects of air pollution (see page 164). Nevertheless, most affected children have allergic asthma, often associated with eczema or hay fever. The most commonly recognised provoking factor is the house-dust mite, and measures to reduce exposure to this allergen may reduce the severity of asthma[5].

Ninety per cent of general practices now offer supervision of asthma under the Chronic Disease Management Programme, and patients are taught self-management based on measurement of peak expiratory flow-rate (PEFR) and frequency of symptoms. During 1993, the British Thoracic Society published revised guidelines[6] for the management of asthma, which were recommended as guidance by the NHS Management Executive when planning contracts for the care of patients with asthma[7]. The emphasis is on regular anti-inflammatory treatment and stepwise increases in medication, as required, to control symptoms and to maintain the best possible PEFRs. The guidelines also suggest criteria for referral and admission to hospital, and for discharge. Patients with asthma who have had previous life-threatening attacks or who have been admitted to hospital within the past 12 months appear to be at particular risk of a severe attack, and the need for ambulance staff and triage nurses in accident and emergency departments to start treatment without delay has been emphasised[8].

The Chronic Disease Management Programme specifies that clinics should be run by staff with appropriate training and the National Asthma Training Centre has given a valuable lead in training nurses in primary and hospital care. The National Asthma Task Force, which is supported by DH, is assessing trends in asthma mortality, as well as optimum therapy and organisation of care.

References

1. Anderson HR, Esmail A, Hollowell J, Littlejohns P, Strachan D. *Lower Respiratory Disease*. In: Stevens A, Raftery J, eds. *Health Care Needs Assessment*, vol 1. Oxford: Radcliffe Medical Press (in press).
2. Shaw RA, Crane J, O'Donnell TV, Porteous LE, Colman ED. Increasing asthma prevalence in a rural New Zealand population 1975-89. *Arch Dis Child* 1990; **65**: 1319-23.
3. Aberg N. Asthma and allergic rhinitis in Swedish conscripts. *Clin Exp Allergy* 1989; **19**: 59-63.
4. Arshad SH, Hide DW. Effect of environmental factors on the development of allergic disorders in infancy. *J Allergy Clin Immunol* 1992; **90**: 235-41.
5. Colloff MJ, Ayres J, Carswell F et al. BSACI Working Group on Control of Domestic Allergens: the control of allergens of dust mites and domestic pets: a position paper. *Clin Exp Allergy* 1992; **22 (Suppl 2)**: 1-28.
6. British Thoracic Society. Guidelines on the management of asthma. *Thorax* 1993; **48 (Suppl 2)**: S1-S24.
7. Department of Health. *Improving Clinical Effectiveness*. Heywood (Lancashire): Department of Health, 1993 (Executive Letter: EL(93)115).
8. Richards GN, Kolbe J, Genwick J, Ree HH. Demographic characteristics of patients with severe life-threatening asthma: comparison with asthma deaths. *Thorax* 1993; **48**: 1105-9.

(f)   Osteopathy and chiropractic

After a Private Peer's Bill to regulate osteopathy fell in 1992 when Parliament was prorogued for the general election, Mr Malcolm Moss MP successfully introduced a Private Member's Bill on Osteopathy, which received Royal Assent in July[1]. The main purpose of the Act is to establish a General Osteopathic Council to regulate, develop and promote the profession of osteopathy and to ensure that only those persons who are suitably qualified both personally and professionally, and who are registered under the statutory scheme, are allowed to practise as, and call themselves, osteopaths. The General Osteopathic Council - and four statutory committees to cover education, investigation, professional conduct, and health - is now being set up.

Following the publication in May of the King's Fund Working Party report on chiropractic, Mr David Lidington MP introduced into the House of Commons a Private Member's Bill, modelled on the *Osteopathy Act*[1], to regulate chiropractic; it has received all-Party support and is likely to receive its Second Reading early in 1994.

There are about 2,500 osteopaths and 900 chiropractors in the UK, most of whom work in private practice, although fundholding GPs, for example, can use part of their NHS budgets to employ complementary therapists on a sessional basis[2]. In December, a 2-year research project was commissioned from the Medical Care Research Unit at the University of Sheffield to assess the impact that osteopaths, chiropractors and other complementary therapists have on other aspects of health care within general practice.

References

1. *Osteopathy Act 1993*. London: HMSO, 1993.
2. Bingham T. *Report of a Working Party on Chiropractic*. London: King Edward's Hospital Fund for London, 1993. Chair: Sir Thomas Bingham.

(g)   Mental health

(i)   *Mental health and primary care*

Primary care provides considerable opportunities to achieve the mental health targets of the Health of the Nation initiative[1] (see page 65) and several projects are now under way[2,3]. DH, the Royal College of General Practitioners (RCGP), the Mental Health Foundation and the Gatsby Charitable Foundation have established a senior RCGP Fellowship in continuing mental health education in primary care, and the role of GP facilitators in mental health is being evaluated. Simple strategies in which practice nurses use agreed protocols may greatly improve patients' compliance with treatment, and a study to assess the role of practice nurses in the treatment of depression has been set up. A further project evaluates a 'model' general practice to develop the best possible care for patients with depression, anxiety, somatisation, schizophrenia and alcohol misuse. The NHS Management Executive has funded the University of Exeter to develop audit of the quality of primary care for depression.

DH also provides financial and technical support for the professional and public education initiatives of the 'Defeat Depression' campaign organised by the Royal College of Psychiatrists and the RCGP.

(ii)   *Occupational mental health*

Poor mental health not only causes suffering to individuals but also has a major impact on employers and the economy as a whole. Approximately one in every ten adults suffers from some form of mental ill-health every year, at a cost to British industry of at least £3.7 billion annually. For every working day lost because of industrial disputes in the United Kingdom (UK) during 1989/90, 20 were lost due to effects of mental illness. In 1991, 91.5 million days of certified sickness absence were caused by mental ill-health in the UK; the true total figure for psychiatric morbidity may well be higher due to some employees' reluctance to let their employers or even their doctors know about depression or other mental illness.

In conjunction with the Confederation of British Industry (CBI), the Health and Safety Executive (HSE), the Health Education Authority (HEA) and other organisations, DH held a conference in January on 'Promoting mental health policies in the workplace' which was addressed by the Secretary of State for Health. The conference proceedings were published in August[4].

As part of the Public Information Strategy, DH also published a booklet for employers, *A Guide to Mental Health in the Workplace*[5] which explains the effects of mental ill-health at work and describes actions which can help to improve employees' mental health. The booklet was launched at the annual conference of the Institute of Personnel Management, and DH also sponsored a stand on this theme at the annual CBI conference in November.

Mental health of the NHS workforce is one of six NHS research and development priorities in mental health and various studies have been commissioned.

(iii)   *Services for people with severe mental illness*

In January, the Secretary of State for Health established a Working Group to review legal powers on the care of mentally ill people in the community. Its report was published in August[6], and concluded that, although the Mental Health Act 1983[7] contains powers which provide for most eventualities they are not always used to greatest effect, and that a power of supervised discharge should supplement them. Such a power would, for those made subject to it, provide a statutory framework for the care programme approach. A treatment plan would be negotiated and, if the patient subsequently failed to comply with it, his or her key worker would call an immediate review to consider whether the patient had deteriorated to the extent that criteria for compulsory admission to hospital programme were met, or whether alternative strategies were needed.

The improvement of care for severely mentally ill people involves a comprehensive package of measures and the Secretary of State for Health also announced a plan to develop safe and successful community care[8]. Other initiatives include: publication of a revised Code of Practice for the Mental Health Act 1983[7]; guidance on discharge; better training for key workers under the care programme approach; a CSAG review of standards of care for people with schizophrenia; an agreed work programme for the Mental Health Task Force; steps to ensure that health authority and GP fundholder purchasing plans cover the essential needs for mental health services; an action plan to improve mental health services in London; and the development of better information systems, including supervision registers.

The teams set up under the Homeless Mentally Ill Initiative[9] continued their work with severely mentally ill people sleeping rough or in hostels, and a further 149 places in hostels were made available in inner London. The Mental Illness Specific Grant funded 800 schemes that covered 64,000 people.

(iv)   *Services for mentally disordered offenders*

Following the completion of a joint DH/Home Office review of health and social services for mentally disordered offenders[10,11], further reports on service needs in the community, hospital and prison[12]; finance, staffing and training[13]; academic development and research[14]; and special issues and differing needs[15] were published early in 1993. Ministers have accepted that services should, as resources allow, develop along the lines proposed by the review. Awareness of the severity and diversity of the needs of mentally disordered offenders has been greatly improved by the review and the work arising from it, and the topic was identified in last year's Report as a key issue[10]. A second national needs assessment exercise[16], co-ordinated by RDsPH, involved the NHS, the prison service and the Special Hospitals Service Authority. NHS priorities and planning guidance for 1994/95[17] identifies services for mentally disordered offenders as a first-order priority, and requires health authorities to work with social services and criminal justice agencies to develop strategic and purchasing plans to meet the needs of this group, including transferred or discharged prisoners, and to ensure the placement within six months of special hospital patients who no longer need high security care.

A fully integrated service for mentally disordered offenders requires multi-agency working between the NHS, social services and criminal justice agencies (including prisons, and assessment and diversion arrangements), and application of the care programme approach[18] to people discharged from hospital and those released from prison. The special needs of people with mild to moderate learning disabilities, who often fall through the network of care, were highlighted in the review[19] and by a working group chaired by Professor James Mansell[20].

Service development has been aided by additional central funding for medium-secure services to provide a total of over 650 beds; the original target[21] will be

Figure 5.2: *Transfers to hospital from prison under Sections 47/48 of Mental Health Act 1983, England and Wales, 1984-93*

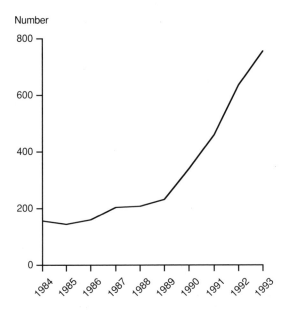

Source: Home Office Statistical Bulletin

exceeded by 1995. Pump-priming money has helped to promote 37 local multi-agency schemes in 1993, and funding from the Home Office has helped to establish court assessment and diversion schemes. Transfers to hospital from prison of those requiring inpatient care have risen from 103 in 1982 to 755 in 1993 (an 18.9% increase from the previous year; see Figure 5.2).

(v)   Mental health legislation

Previous Reports[22,23,24,25,26] have drawn attention to the difficulties in ensuring effective and safe care outside hospital for some mentally disordered people. An official review team was established to consider, among other matters, whether new legal powers were needed to ensure that mentally ill people in the community get the care they need, and whether the present legal powers in the Mental Health Act 1983[7] were being used as effectively as they should be and what action could be taken to ensure that they are. The team's report, published in August[6], recommended that the 1983 Act should be amended to provide for supervised discharge of non-restricted patients who have been detained in hospital and who would present a serious risk unless their care was supervised. The Secretary of State for Health has announced her intention to introduce such legislation.

References

1.   Department of Health. *The Health of the Nation: a strategy for health in England*. London: HMSO, 1992 (Cm. 1986).
2.   Department of Health. *The Health of the Nation: one year on - a report on the progress of the Health of the Nation*. London: HMSO, 1993: 80-5.
3.   Jenkins R. Developments in the primary care of mental illness: a forward look. *Int Rev Psychiatry* 1992: **4**: 237-43.
4.   Jenkins R, Warman D. *Promoting mental health policies in the workplace*. London: HMSO, 1993.
5.   Department of Health. *Mental Illness: a guide to mental health in the workplace*. London: Department of Health, 1993.
6.   Department of Health. *Legal powers on the care of mentally ill people in the community*. London: Department of Health, 1993.
7.   *Mental Health Act 1983*. London: HMSO, 1983.
8.   Department of Health. *Legislation planned to provide for supervised discharge of psychiatric patients*. London: Department of Health, 1993 (Press Release: H93/908).
9.   Department of Health. *On the State of the Public Health: the annual report of the Chief Medical Officer of the Department of Health for the year 1992*. London: HMSO, 1993; 120.
10. Department of Health. *On the State of the Public Health: the annual report of the Chief Medical Officer of the Department of Health for the year 1992*. London: HMSO, 1993: 122-3.
11. Department of Health, Home Office. *Review of health and social services for mentally disordered offenders and others requiring similar services: final summary report*. London: HMSO, 1992 (Cm. 2088).
12. Department of Health, Home Office. *Review of health and social services for mentally disordered offenders and others requiring similar services: volume 2: service needs: the reports of the community, hospital and prison advisory groups and an overview by the steering committee*. London: HMSO, 1993. Chair: Dr John Reed.
13. Department of Health, Home Office. *Review of health and social services for mentally disordered offenders and others requiring similar services: volume 3: finance, staffing and training: the reports of the finance and staffing and training advisory groups*. London: HMSO, 1993. Chair: Dr John Reed.
14. Department of Health, Home Office. *Review of health and social services for mentally disordered offenders and others requiring similar services: volume 4: the reports of the academic and research base: the reports of the academic development and research advisory groups*. London: HMSO, 1993. Chair: Dr John Reed.
15. Department of Health, Home Office. *Review of health and social services for mentally disordered offenders and others requiring similar services: volume 5: special issues and differing needs: the report of the official working group on services for people with special needs*. London: HMSO, 1993. Chair: Dr John Reed.
16. Department of Health. *Assessment of need for services for mentally disordered offenders and others with similar needs*. Heywood (Lancashire): Department of Health, 1993 (Executive Letter: EL(93)68).
17. NHS Management Executive. *Priorities and planning guidance 1994/95*. Heywood (Lancashire): Department

of Health, 1993 (Executive Letter: EL(93)54).

18. Department of Health. *The care programme approach for people with a mental illness referred to the specialist psychiatric service.* Heywood (Lancashire): Department of Health, 1990 (Health Circular: HC(90)23, Local Authority Social Services Letter: LASSL(90)11).

19. Department of Health, Home Office. *Review of services for mentally disordered offenders and others requiring similar services: vol 7: people with learning disabilities (mental disability) or autism.* London: HMSO (in press).

20. Department of Health. *Services for people with learning disabilities and challenging behaviour or mental health needs: report of a project group.* London: HMSO, 1992. Chair: Professor James Mansell.

21. Department of Health and Social Security. *Revised Report of the Working Party on Security in NHS Psychiatric Hospitals.* London: Department of Health and Social Security, 1974.

22. Department of Health and Social Security. *On the State of the Public Health: the annual report of the Chief Medical Officer of the Department of Health and Social Security for the year 1987.* London: HMSO, 1988; 71-3.

23. Department of Health. *On the State of the Public Health: the annual report of the Chief Medical Officer of the Department of Health for the year 1988.* London: HMSO, 1989; 174-5.

24. Department of Health. *On the State of the Public Health: the annual report of the Chief Medical Officer of the Department of Health for the year 1989.* London: HMSO, 1990; 130-1.

25. Department of Health. *On the State of the Public Health: the annual report of the Chief Medical Officer of the Department of Health for the year 1990.* London: HMSO, 1991; 170-1.

26. Department of Health. *On the State of the Public Health: the annual report of the Chief Medical Officer of the Department of Health for the year 1991.* London: HMSO, 1992; 120.

(h)   Maternity and child health services

(i)   *Report of the Expert Maternity Group*

The Report[1] for 1992 indicated that an Expert Maternity Group had been set up under the chairmanship of Baroness Cumberlege, Parliamentary Under Secretary of State for Health in the House of Lords. The Group's terms of reference were "to review policy on NHS maternity care, particularly during childbirth, and to make recommendations" and its report, *Changing Childbirth*[2], was published for consultation in August 1993. It included the results of a survey of communications practice in maternity services[3].

The principle which underpins the proposals in the report is that the mother and her baby should be at the centre of all planning and provision of maternity care. The report recognised a need for the mother to be an active partner in decisions that affect her care and for professionals to support her in this. Good communication about all available services, including unbiased information about the advantages and disadvantages of each option, was seen to be essential to enable the mother to exercise choice. Furthermore, there ought to be greater continuity of care and carer to promote security and confidence. In addition to the established Patient's Charter[4] principle that every woman should have a named midwife, the Group identified a need for a lead professional to give a substantial part of the care; for an uncomplicated pregnancy, this person would usually be the named midwife.

The report recognised the need for substantial changes in professional practice to secure a woman-centred service. However, such changes should help to ensure greater accessibility and acceptability of maternity care. It is essential to provide the safest practicable service at birth, wherever that takes place, and whenever possible maternity services should be founded on clinical practices of known effectiveness[5]. Responses to the consultation will be considered carefully before any arrangements are made to implement the report's recommendations.

(ii)   Confidential Enquiries into Maternal Deaths

The Report of the Confidential Enquiries into Maternal Deaths in the United Kingdom 1988-1990 was prepared during the year and will be published early in 1994[6]. Findings show that the maternal mortality rate has remained essentially unchanged, at 10 per 100,000 maternities, since the Report for 1985-1987[7]. The most common causes of direct maternal death remained thrombosis and thromboembolism, hypertensive disorders of pregnancy, haemorrhage and ectopic pregnancy, which together accounted for over 60% of deaths.

The Report will include recommendations on clinical care, including guidelines on the management of massive haemorrhage and on the provision of maternity services.

(iii)   Folic acid and neural tube defects

Following the report of an expert advisory group in 1992[8], the Chief Medical and Nursing Officers issued guidance[9] to advise all women who were planning to conceive that they should increase their folic acid intake by dietary means and through food supplements. Doses of 5 mg daily were recommended to prevent recurrence, and 0.4 mg daily to prevent a first occurrence, of a neural tube defect (NTD) in the foetus. During 1993, copies of this report and the professional guidance were distributed widely and DH also prepared a leaflet and poster for public education. During the year there has been increasing availability of folic acid food supplements at the lower dose.

(iv)   Vitamin A and pregnancy

The Committee on Toxicity of Chemicals in Food, Consumer Products and the Environment (COT) recently reviewed the results of a study in young women which compared the concentrations of vitamin A and its metabolites in the blood after eating liver with those found after an equivalent amount of vitamin A was taken as dietary supplements. It had been thought that fewer potentially teratogenic metabolites might be absorbed after eating liver than after taking dietary supplements, but this was not the case. The Chief Medical Officer confirmed[10] earlier advice to health professionals that women who are pregnant or who might become pregnant should not consume excessive amounts of liver or vitamin A supplements.

(v)   Human Fertilisation and Embryology Authority

The Human Fertilisation and Embryology Authority (HFEA), chaired by Sir Colin Campbell, was set up in 1990 under the provisions of the Human Fertilisation and Embryology Act 1990[11]. It is responsible for the regulation of

131

clinical practice that involves the creation or keeping of human embryos outwith a woman's body, the donation and cryopreservation of gametes, and research on embryos. Regulation is achieved by licensing and a Code of Practice[12].

The work done by the HFEA is widely respected and its licensing system is effective. The Authority has addressed contentious ethical issues by seeking public responses to consultation documents. During 1993, consultations about sex selection[13] led to the conclusion that such techniques were only appropriate for medical, not social, reasons. Preparation of a consultation document on the use of donated ovarian tissue in embryo research and assisted conception is now under way.

(vi)   Sudden infant death syndrome

As anticipated in last year's Report[14], the extended report of the Chief Medical Officer's Expert Group on the Sleeping Position of Infants and Cot Death was published during 1993[15]. Although some of the evidence was not available when the Group gave its initial advice in 1991[16], it found no reason to modify its views except in detail and emphasis. The recommendations were that, except in particular circumstances and on medical advice, the great majority of infants should be nursed on their backs; that infants should not be exposed to cigarette smoke either before birth or afterwards, and that parents and prospective parents should be advised of this risk; and that guidance on infant care should incorporate a number of points related to room temperature, bedding and sources of heat. The Group also recommended that breast-feeding be encouraged wherever possible, whilst recognising that the evidence from published studies does not consistently show that breast-feeding affects the risk of cot death, and that those entrusted with the care of infants should be encouraged to seek medical advice promptly if an infant is unwell or thought to be unwell. A summary of the evidence and the Group's conclusions and recommendations was sent to health professionals by the Chief Medical and Nursing Officers[17].

These changes in infant care will not eliminate sudden infant death syndrome (SIDS), which will not be possible until the underlying causes and the processes leading to such deaths are fully understood, but they will reduce the risk of cot death. The Group recommended further biomedical and health services research into SIDS and other infant deaths of unknown cause, and noted the need to monitor the effects of recommended interventions. Preliminary data on the incidence of SIDS in 1993 indicate that the low level recorded in 1992 has been maintained.

(vii)   Prophylaxis of vitamin K deficiency bleeding in infants

The Report for 1992[18] drew attention to concerns about the use of vitamin K in the prevention of vitamin K deficiency bleeding in infants, in particular a reported association between vitamin K given intramuscularly and childhood cancer[19,20,21], and described action that had been taken during the year. In 1993, DH commissioned research studies in the UK to investigate the reported association, to monitor local policy and practice in vitamin K prophylaxis, and to determine the incidence and circumstances of haemorrhagic disease in infants.

Meanwhile, studies in Sweden[22] and the United States of America (USA)[23] were unable to verify any association between vitamin K and childhood cancer, but the estimates of relative risk showed wide confidence intervals and were not conclusive. Any possible carcinogenic effects of vitamin K should be identified by the larger studies now under way[24]. In view of continued concern among health professionals and parents, and the difficulties that have arisen because of different clinical practices, a review of vitamin K prophylaxis will be carried out during 1994.

(viii)   Neonatal intensive care

In July 1993, the Clinical Standards Advisory Group (CSAG) published its first report, *Access to and Availability of Specialist Services*[25], which encompassed the reports of four separate Working Groups. One of these groups, convened by Professor Sir David Hull, was set up to consider neonatal intensive care (NIC)[26] and collected a great deal of information not previously available or brought together. Its report contained the following recommendations:

- NIC services should be planned for groups of Districts or at Regional level according to population and geography;

- a managed market is needed to ensure adequate provision and to maximise efficiency;

- each DHA should calculate its needs to purchase NIC, and quality and quantity should be specified;

- purchasing authorities should form consortia to purchase NIC, and provider units should be encouraged through contracts to work closely together, sharing resources if appropriate;

- contracts should be based on a small and agreed range of diagnostic and therapeutic groupings;

- senior clinical staff should be involved in the contract process and all clinical staff kept fully informed; *and*

- all NIC units should be appraised against national standards of service provision.

In its response[27], the Government observed that many of these points were common to other specialised services: they included the need for DHAs to join together for planning and purchasing; the inadequacies of block contracts; the case for a managed market; and the value of national criteria to appraise services. The Government's response also noted that the care of all small and seriously ill babies in need of intensive care facilities in any given District or Region has always been a challenge for the health service. The task now is to ensure that this challenge is effectively tackled through the purchasing system. The Government recognised the need for providers to work closely together to facilitate the placement of ill babies, with mechanisms to monitor the extent to which unmet needs are being identified and addressed. The CSAG study also showed that improvements need to be made to the methods of costing NIC services, and its suggestions would be considered.

(ix) Paediatric intensive care

The report of a multidisciplinary working party on paediatric intensive care, convened by the British Paediatric Association, was published in November[28]. It was underpinned by the most detailed survey of the care of critically ill children ever conducted in the UK. This survey, which was funded by DH, revealed an uneven provision of paediatric intensive care services across the country and expressed concern that some children may not receive the care that they need from nurses and doctors who were trained and had experience in paediatric intensive care. The Minister for Health welcomed the report, and asked the NHS Management Executive to ensure that health authorities were aware of the report and made a co-ordinated and effective response to extend existing facilities and training programmes[29].

(x) Confidential Enquiry into Stillbirths and Deaths in Infancy

Following the work described in the 1992 Report[30], the first year's programme for the Confidential Enquiry into Stillbirths and Deaths in Infancy (CESDI) was implemented from 1 January 1993. Good progress was made during the year, with the establishment of a reporting network and Regional confidential enquiry panels. A rapid reporting system enabled data collection on all deaths in babies or infants from 20 weeks of gestation to one year-of-age. Confidential enquiries were conducted on normally formed babies with a birthweight of at least 2.5 kg who died during or shortly after labour, and on sudden unexpected infant deaths (including cot deaths). In addition, a case control study into sudden unexpected infant deaths was started in South Western and Yorkshire RHAs in February, with the inclusion of Trent RHA in September. The importance of post-mortem investigations to establish the causes of unexpected infant deaths was recognised by the production of information about such examinations for bereaved parents[31], and the development of an audit procedure for CESDI pathology guidelines: these were included in a booklet on post-mortem investigations issued by the Royal College of Pathologists in August[32].

The National Advisory Body (NAB), under the chairmanship of Lady Littler, steers and guides CESDI with the support of a secretariat in DH. In 1993, additional work was conducted by two NAB working groups on statistics and epidemiology, and on pathology. The NAB Annual Report[33], submitted to Ministers in November, contained a summary of the methods used by CESDI and provisional results from the rapid reporting system. During 1993, several workshops were held for CESDI regional co-ordinators. They supplemented guidelines distributed by the NAB secretariat, who also produced a quarterly newsletter for circulation to co-ordinators, clinicians and others with an interest in CESDI. The NAB agreed on a broadly similar programme for 1994, with an extension of the intrapartum-related confidential enquiries to babies of lower birthweight (from 1.5 kg), a case-control study of antepartum deaths in selected Regions, as well as work to evaluate the confidential enquiry panels and other aspects of CESDI. The results of the 1993 enquiries and data derived from the rapid reporting system will be presented to Ministers in the NAB's next Annual Report, due to be published towards the end of 1994.

(xi)   Notification of congenital malformations

The OPCS notification system to monitor congenital malformations was introduced in 1964 after the outbreak of phocomelia associated with ingestion of thalidomide during pregnancy. It was established to provide an early warning system for the detection of any increase in the incidence of malformations identified at or within seven days of birth - later extended to ten days. Although the system was set up primarily to monitor change, it now represents an extensive database of the prevalence of congenital malformations in England and Wales. Nevertheless, the existing system has recognised deficiencies. It specifies the reporting of malformations, rather than other types of congenital defect or anomaly, and only accepts notifications of those babies whose malformations are observed within ten days of birth. Some Districts fail to notify malformations in stillborn infants; some malformations in neonatal deaths may be overlooked; babies born outside their mother's home health District may not be notified; there is no systematic audit of the completeness or timeliness of ascertainment or validation of the diagnosis; and there is no mechanism to notify revisions or to update published data.

A comparison of 1991 notification data with equivalent data from certifications of stillbirths and neonatal deaths showed that only 80% of notifications could be matched with corresponding death registrations, and that only 40% of infant deaths in which congenital malformation was mentioned on the death certificate could be matched with a notification. In view of these deficiencies, and the need to ensure early detection of congenital anomalies as well as malformations, and to monitor for abnormalities that occur earlier in pregnancy and later in infancy, the Medical Advisory Committee of the Registrar General set up a Working Group to review the operation of the national system and how it might be expanded to include these other factors. The Group will take into account the introduction of the new OPCS information technology strategy; developments in diagnosis, coding and statistical analysis; the need for quality control; and the paramount constraints of confidentiality and data protection. The Working Group is expected to report in 1994.

(xii)   *Gene Therapy Advisory Committee*

During 1993, the Secretary of State for Health established a new non-statutory body, the Gene Therapy Advisory Committee (GTAC)[34,35,36], to succeed the Committee on the Ethics of Gene Therapy (CEGT; see page 185).

GTAC, chaired by Professor Dame June Lloyd, brings together a wide range of medical, scientific, legal, ethical and lay expertise. Its remit includes consideration of all proposals for gene therapy research on human subjects in the UK and to provide advice on their acceptability on ethical grounds, taking account of the scientific merits and the potential benefits and risks. The Committee met for the first time in November.

During 1993, under the transitional arrangements operated by CEGT, the first three UK gene therapy research trials gained ethical approval - a therapeutic trial of gene replacement therapy in a child with severe combined immunodeficiency syndrome caused by adenosine deaminase deficiency, and preliminary trials in patients with cystic fibrosis and B-cell lymphoma. By the end of the year, GTAC had four more proposals under consideration; these cover research on malignant melanoma, neuroblastoma and cystic fibrosis.

The rapid scientific advances in genetic research offer the prospect that an increasing range of human diseases may benefit from the use of gene therapy. However, it is essential that the first steps in gene therapy research in patients are governed by a stringent code of practice, not only to establish the precise effectiveness of such procedures but also to ensure a full ethical review of the merit, acceptability and safety of each research proposal.

References

1. Department of Health. *On the State of the Public Health: the annual report of the Chief Medical Officer of the Department of Health for the year 1992.* London: HMSO, 1993; 125.
2. Department of Health. *Changing Childbirth: part 1: report of the Expert Maternity Group.* London: HMSO, 1993. Chair: Baroness Cumberlege.
3. Department of Health. *Changing Childbirth: part 2: survey of good communications practice in maternity services.* London: HMSO, 1993. Chair: Baroness Cumberlege.
4. Department of Health. *The Patient's Charter.* London: Department of Health, 1991.
5. Enkin M, Keirse M, Chalmers I. *Effective Care in Pregnancy and Childbirth.* Oxford: Oxford University Press, 1989.
6. Department of Health, Welsh Office, Scottish Home and Health Department, Northern Ireland Department of Health and Social Services. *Report on Confidential Enquiries into Maternal Deaths in the United Kingdom 1988-90.* London: HMSO (in press).
7. Department of Health, Welsh Office, Scottish Home and Health Department, Northern Ireland Department of Health and Social Services. *Report on Confidential Enquiries into Maternal Deaths in the United Kingdom 1985-1987.* London: HMSO, 1991.
8. Department of Health. *Folic acid and the prevention of neural tube defects.* Heywood (Lancashire): Department of Health, 1992. Chair: Dame June Lloyd.
9. Department of Health. *Folic acid and the prevention of neural tube defects: guidelines on prevention.* London: Department of Health, 1992 (Professional Letter: PL/CMO(92)18, PL/CNO(92)12).
10. Department of Health. *Vitamin A and pregnancy.* Heywood (Lancashire): Department of Health, 1993 (Professional Letter: PL/CMO(93)15).
11. *Human Fertilisation and Embryology Act 1990.* London: HMSO, 1990.
12. *Human Fertilisation and Embryology Authority Code of Practice (Revised 1993).* London: Human Fertilisation and Embryology Authority, 1993.
13. Human Fertilisation and Embryology Authority. *Sex Selection: public consultation document.* London: Human Fertilisation and Embryology Authority, 1993.
14. Department of Health. *On the State of the Public Health: the annual report of the Chief Medical Officer of the*

Department of Health for the year 1992. London: HMSO, 1993; 129-30.

15. Department of Health. *Report of the Chief Medical Officer's Expert Group on the Sleeping Position of Infants and Cot Death*. London: HMSO, 1993. Chair: Dr Eileen Rubery.

16. Department of Health. *How to reduce the risk of cot deaths*. London: Department of Health, 1991 (Press Release: H91/514).

17. Department of Health. *Cot Death*. Heywood (Lancashire): Department of Health, 1993 (Professional Letter: PL/CMO(93)4, PL/CNO(93)3).

18. Department of Health. *On the State of the Public Health: the annual report of the Chief Medical Officer of the Department of Health for the year 1992*. London: HMSO, 1993: 130-1.

19. Golding J, Birmingham K, Greenwood R, Mott M. Childhood cancer, intramuscular vitamin K, and pethidine given during labour. *BMJ* 1992; **305**: 341-6.

20. Draper GJ, Stiller CA. Intramuscular vitamin K and childhood cancer. *BMJ* 1992; **305**: 709.

21. Hull D. Vitamin K and childhood cancer. The risk of haemorrhagic disease is certain; that of cancer is not. *BMJ* 1992; **305**: 326-7.

22. Ekelund H, Finnstrom O, Gunnarskog J, Kallen B, Larsson Y. Administration of vitamin K to newborn infants and childhood cancer. *BMJ* 1993; **307**: 89-91.

23. Klebanoff MA, Read JS, Mills JL, Shiono PH. The risk of childhood cancer after neonatal exposure to vitamin K. *N Engl J Med* 1993; **329**: 905-8.

24. Passmore SJ, Draper GJ, Stiller CA. Vitamin K and childhood cancer. *BMJ* 1993; **307**: 1140.

25. Clinical Standards Advisory Group. *Access to and Availability of Specialist Services: report of a CSAG committee*. London: HMSO, 1993. Chair: Professor John Richmond.

26. Department of Health. *Neonatal Intensive Care: access to and availability of specialist services: report of a CSAG working group*. London: HMSO, 1993. Chair: Professor Sir David Hull.

27. Department of Health. *Government response to the reports by the Clinical Standards Advisory Group on access to and availability of specialist services*. London: Department of Health, 1993.

28. British Paediatric Association. *The Care of Critically Ill Children: report of the multidisciplinary working party on paediatric intensive care convened by the British Paediatric Association*. London: British Paediatric Association, 1993.

29. House of Commons. Parliamentary Debate. Paediatric intensive care. Hansard 24 November 1993; **233**: Col 453-8.

30. Department of Health. *On the State of the Public Health: the annual report of the Chief Medical Officer of the Department of Health for the year 1992*. London: HMSO, 1993.

31. National Advisory Body for the Confidential Enquiry into Stillbirths and Deaths in Infancy. *Guide to the Post-Mortem Examination: brief notes for parents and families who have lost a baby in pregnancy or early infancy*. London: Department of Health, 1993.

32. Royal College of Pathologists. *Guidelines for Post-mortem Reports*. London: Royal College of Pathologists, 1993.

33. National Advisory Body on the Confidential Enquiry into Stillbirths and Deaths in Infancy, Department of Health. *Report: March 1992-July 1993*. London: Department of Health, 1993. Chair: Lady Littler.

34. Department of Health. *New committee to consider proposals for the use of gene therapy*. London: Department of Health, 1993 (Press Release: H93/566).

35 Department of Health. *Professor of child health appointed to chair new Gene Therapy Advisory Committee*. London: Department of Health, 1993 (Press Release: H93/767).

36. Department of Health. *Appointment of Members of the Gene Therapy Advisory Committee*. London: Department of Health, 1993 (Press Release: H93/1056).

(i)   Learning disabilities

The requirements of people with learning disabilities who have behavioural disturbance or mental health needs has to be taken into account when developing policy for community care. A Project Group, chaired by Professor James Mansell, published its report *Services for People with Learning Disabilities and Challenging Behaviour or Mental Health Needs*[1], in February. Conferences were held in London and in Leeds to mark its launch, and copies of the report were sent to health[2] and local authorities[3]. An Advisory Group, chaired by Mr Andrew McCulloch, and a National Implementation Network were set up to encourage and oversee progress.

The Advisory Group is currently reviewing the use of NHS review processes to encourage implementation of the report, the costs of the required services, the role of psychiatric specialists in learning disability, and the need for more detailed guidance for purchasers of health care. DH has funded the Tizard Centre (formerly the Centre for Applied Psychology of Social Care) at the University of Kent to establish an implementation network. Dissemination of information about good practice, facilitation of information exchange, and feedback from local initiatives should help in the planning and provision of care. DH's Social Security Inspectorate commissioned the Association for Residential Care and the National Association for the Protection from Sexual Abuse of Adults and Children with Learning Disabilities to investigate the prevention and treatment of sexual abuse of adults with learning disabilities in residential care; their report[4] was published in November and circulated to all directors of social services.

The NHS Management Executive published a booklet[5] on learning disabilities to encourage purchasers to take into account patients' points of view when commissioning general health services for people with learning disabilities.

References

1. Department of Health. *Services for People with Learning Disabilities and Challenging Behaviour or Mental Health Needs: report of a project group.* London: HMSO, 1993. Chair: Professor James Mansell.
2. Department of Health. *Services for People with Learning Disabilities and Challenging Behaviour or Mental Health Needs: report of a project group.* Leeds: NHS Management Executive, 1993.
3. Department of Health. *Mansell Report on Services for People with Learning Disabilities and Challenging Behaviour or Mental Health Needs.* Heywood (Lancashire): Department of Health, 1993 (Local Authority Social Services Letter: LASSL(93)1).
4. Association for Residential Care, National Association for the Protection from Sexual Abuse of Adults and Children with Learning Disabilities (NAPSAC). *It Could Never Happen Here: the prevention and treatment of sexual abuse of adults with learning disabilities in residential settings.* Nottingham: NAPSAC, 1993.
5. Department of Health. *Learning disabilities.* Leeds: NHS Management Executive, 1993.

(j)   Disability and rehabilitation

During 1993, there were further developments in the fields of disability, rehabilitation and audiology.

In March, the Public Accounts Committee of the House of Commons considered the National Audit Office report on health services for physically disabled people aged 16 to 64 years[1]. Its own report, published in December[2], expressed concern that many health authorities lack up-to-date information on the numbers and needs of disabled people; it highlighted the importance of developing targets for this complex but important range of services. The findings indicated that some disabled people were unclear about where they should apply for services; and that some may be discharged from hospital into the community without adequate arrangements for continuity of care. The length of time taken to deliver wheelchairs and other aids was identified as a matter for concern, as was availability of effective services for people with urinary incontinence. The incidence of pressure sores among hospital inpatients was also felt to be too high.

In June, the Chief Executive of the NHS Management Executive set out priorities for the NHS for 1994/95[3], and asked RHAs to ensure that services for physically disabled people met local standards in all Districts according to assessments of need and after consultation with disabled people and their carers. In association with CSAG, DH held a conference in May on pressure sores; at the end of the year DH published *Pressure Sores: a key quality indicator*[4] to assist purchasers and providers of health care services.

There were other worthwhile achievements during 1993. The Advisory Group on Rehabilitation met on four occasions. DH's initiative to improve NHS rehabilitation facilities for people who had suffered brain injury, announced in 1992, was fully established. Bids were invited for research to develop measurable targets relevant to the development of NHS services for physically disabled people. An Advisory Group on research and development priorities for people with physical and complex disabilities provided advice to the NHS Central Research and Development Committee. Towards the end of 1993, a report on medical education on disability was published[5]. A research project on multiple outcome measures to evaluate hearing aid fittings and services was established, in conjunction with the MRC Institute of Hearing Research.

References

1. National Audit Office. *Health Services for Physically Disabled People Aged 16 to 64*. London: HMSO, 1992 (HC 65).
2. House of Commons. *Health Services For Physically Disabled People Aged 16 to 64. 61st Report from the Committee of Public Accounts* (HC 538).
3. Department of Health. *Priorities and planning guidance 1994/95*. Heywood (Lancashire): Department of Health, 1993 (Executive Letter: EL(93)54).
4. Department of Health. *Pressure Sores: a key quality indicator: a guide for NHS purchasers and providers*. Heywood (Lancashire): Department of Health, 1993.
5. Inman C, Kahtan S. Medical education on disability. A report from University College London Medical School and the Prince of Wales Advisory Group on Disability. London: University College London Medical School, 1993.

(k)   Prison health care

The Prison Service became an Executive Agency of the Home Office in April. Its first corporate plan for the three years to the end of March 1996 acknowledged that prisoners have a right to the same range and quality of health care services as the general public and that the Prison Service had to ensure that prisoners' health needs are met either internally, through the Health Care Service for Prisoners, or externally within the NHS or the private sector.

The corporate plan also included specific undertakings about the transfer of mentally disordered prisoners from prison to hospital; the treatment and subsequent support of prisoners who misuse alcohol or drugs; and the need for structured health promotion, and illness prevention programmes, including multidisciplinary programmes to combat HIV infection and AIDS.

Key health objectives for 1993/94 include the delegation of full responsibility for the management of health care services to Governors of individual prisons; the establishment of pilot health promotion programmes at five prisons; the launch of a programme to contract for clinical services; and the extension of hepatitis B immunisation in line with the recommendations of the Joint Committee on Vaccination and Immunisation[1]. A contract for the provision of psychiatric services in North-East England was concluded in June, and in December contracts were offered to two NHS provider units for the provision of genito-urinary medicine services in London. An enhanced hepatitis B immunisation programme was introduced in October and the five health promotion pilot projects were launched in December.

Other research within the Prison Service includes pilot HIV prevalence surveys at three London prisons; pilot work for a national study of prisoners' knowledge, attitudes and behaviour about HIV and AIDS; and preparation for the first national survey of the physical health of prisoners.

Reference

1. Department of Health. *Memorandum "Immunisation against infectious disease"*. Heywood (Lancashire): Department of Health, 1992 (Professional Letter: PL/CMO(92)7).

CHAPTER 6

COMMUNICABLE DISEASES

(a)   HIV infection and AIDS

Government strategy on HIV infection and AIDS

In June, in the light of new projections for HIV infection and AIDS[1], the Government published further details of its strategy on HIV/AIDS. The main aims of this strategy are to ensure that resources and services are properly targeted; that the right balance is struck with other health priorities; and that initiatives to combat HIV infection and AIDS are brought within the mainstream of health care and health promotion.

Progress of the epidemic

AIDS

Surveillance of the epidemic is implemented through the voluntary confidential reporting systems operated by the Public Health Laboratory Service (PHLS) AIDS Centre at the Communicable Disease Surveillance Centre (CDSC)[2,3] and the Government's programme of unlinked anonymous HIV surveys, which is implemented by the PHLS AIDS Centre[4].

The numbers of AIDS cases reported in England are shown in Table 6.1 and Figure 6.1. 1,473 cases of AIDS were reported in England in 1993; these brought the cumulative total of AIDS cases reported since 1982 to 7,890, of whom 5,203 are known to have died. It is estimated that, on average, people newly diagnosed with AIDS were infected with HIV 10 years previously.

In July, the European AIDS surveillance case definition was introduced for use in the United Kingdom (UK).   This adds pulmonary tuberculosis, recurrent pneumonia within twelve months and invasive cervical carcinoma to the list of AIDS-defining diseases in the case surveillance case definition for AIDS used after the 1987 revision of case definition by the United States (US) Centers for Disease Control (CDC). Figure 6.2 compares AIDS reports for Member States of the European Community (EC), and Table 6.2 shows the number of cases and cumulative cases per million population in EC countries.

HIV infection

Table 6.3 and Figure 6.3 show details of reports of newly diagnosed HIV infection in England: a further 2,220 individuals were reported to have HIV infection in England during 1993, bringing the cumulative total of such reports since 1984 to 18,594. However, many factors might influence the decision to be

Table 6.1: *AIDS cases and known deaths by exposure category and date of report, England, 1982-31 December 1993*
(Numbers subject to revision as further data are received or duplicates identified)

How persons probably acquired the virus	Jan 1992-Dec 1992		Jan 1993-Dec 1993		Jan 1982-Dec 1993			
	Cases		Cases		Male		Female	
	Male	Female	Male	Female	Cases	Deaths	Cases	Deaths
Sexual intercourse:								
between men	1008	-	1013	-	6010	4058	-	-
between men and women								
'high risk' partner*	6	17	4	17	25	13	62	34
other partner abroad**	100	71	109	91	417	228	278	126
other partner UK	8	5	16	11	42	21	32	16
under investigation	1	-	2	2	4	3	2	-
Injecting drug use (IDU)	34	15	44	27	187	113	85	51
IDU and sexual intercourse								
between men	23	-	21	-	127	84	-	-
Blood								
Blood factor	42	1	49	-	342	290	5	3
(eg haemophiliacs)								
Blood or tissue transfer								
(eg transfusion)								
Abroad	1	2	3	12	10	4	38	20
UK	2	-	3	2	17	13	18	17
Mother to child	17	9	11	12	45	22	46	24
Other/undetermined	14	4	16	8	80	54	18	9
Total	1256	124	1291	182	7306	4903	584	300

* Men and women who had sex with injecting drug users, or with those infected through blood factor treatment or blood transfusion, and women who had sex with bisexual men.
** Includes persons without other identified risks who are from, or who have lived in, countries where the major route of HIV-1 transmission is through sexual intercourse between men and women.

Source: CDSC

Figure 6.1: *AIDS cases: total numbers and numbers where infection was probably acquired through sexual intercourse between men and women, England, to 31 December 1993*

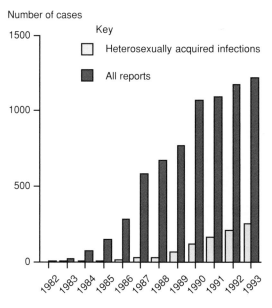

Source: CDSC

Figure 6.2: *Reported AIDS cases in Europe: cumulative rates per million population to December 1993*

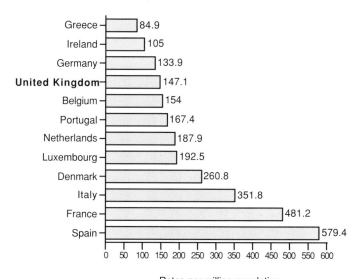

Rates per million population

Source: European Centre for the Epidemiological Monitoring of AIDS

Table 6.2: *AIDS cases reported to WHO by EC countries: cumulative totals at 31 December 1993*

Country	Number of cases	Cumulative cases/ million population
Spain	22655	579.4
France	28497	481.2
Denmark	1356	260.8
Italy	20336	351.8
Netherlands	2912	187.9
Germany*	10858	133.9
Belgium	1555	154.0
Luxembourg	77	192.5
UK	8529	147.1
Portugal	1641	167.4
Ireland	378	105.0
Greece	891	84.9

*Includes the former East Germany.

Source: European Centre for the Epidemiological Monitoring of AIDS

Figure 6.3: *HIV antibody-positive people: total numbers and numbers where infection was probably acquired through sexual intercourse between men and women, England, by year of report to 31 December 1993*

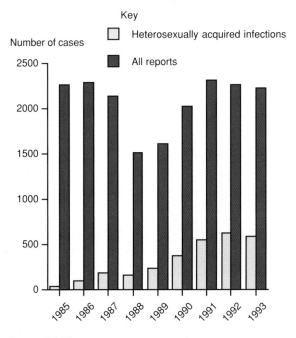

Source: CDSC

Table 6.3: *HIV antibody-positive people by exposure category and date of report, England, to 31 December 1993*
(Numbers subject to revision as further data are received or duplicates identified)

How persons probably acquired the virus	Jan 1992-Dec 1992			Jan 1993-Dec 1993			Nov 1984-Dec 1993		
	Male	Female	NK†	Male	Female	NK†	Male	Female	NK†
Sexual intercourse:									
between men	1338	-	-	1275	-	-	11964	-	-
between men and women									
'high risk' partner*	6	48	-	6	47	-	58	295	-
other partner abroad**	253	253	-	226	213	4	1135	1019	8
other partner UK	12	34	-	18	21	-	67	128	-
under investigation	5	5	-	20	25	-	43	47	-
Injecting drug use (IDU)	115	49	-	102	37	2	1036	472	5
IDU and sexual intercourse									
between men	26	-	-	19	-	-	258	-	-
Blood									
Blood factor (eg haemophiliacs)	9	1	-	4	-	-	1060	10	-
Blood or tissue transfer (eg transfusion)									
Abroad/UK	10	5	-	4	4	-	58	60	1
Mother to child	29	22	-	13	28	1	92	95	1
Other/undetermined	30	6	-	112	33	6	546	101	35
Total	1833	423	-	1799	408	13	16317	2227	50

† NK = Not known (sex not stated on report).

* Men and women who had sex with injecting drug users, or with those infected through blood factor treatment or blood transfusion, and women who had sex with bisexual men.

** Includes persons without other identified risks who are from, or who have lived in, countries where the major route of HIV-1 transmission is through sexual intercourse between men and women.

Source: CDSC

tested for HIV infection, and these reports provide an incomplete indication of the cumulative number of HIV infections since 1984. Evidence of new HIV infection and continued high-risk behaviour among homosexual men[5,6] is of particular concern; men who have sex with men continue to predominate among reports of HIV infection and AIDS.

Unlinked anonymous surveillance

In January 1993, the PHLS published results to mid-1992 from the Government's programme of unlinked anonymous HIV surveys[4]. Preliminary data to mid-1993 indicate that the prevalence of HIV infection among pregnant women in London rose from 1 in 560 in 1990 to 1 in 390 in 1993; the rise was statistically significant in all age-groups.

Unlinked anonymous surveillance in selected genito-urinary medicine (GUM) clinics up to mid-1993 shows an HIV prevalence of 1 in 5 among homosexual men, 1 in 130 among non-drug-injecting heterosexual men and 1 in 160 among non-drug-injecting heterosexual women who attended the participating clinics in London. Outside London, HIV prevalence was 1 in 20 among homosexual men, 1 in 550 among heterosexual men and 1 in 940 among heterosexual women attending GUM clinics.

Comparison of anonymised survey results with the proportion of those tested who were known to be HIV seropositive indicates that a large proportion of people infected with HIV may be unaware of their infection. This proportion is greatest among people who were probably infected through heterosexual sexual intercourse.

AIDS projections

A new report[1] on AIDS projections for England and Wales was published in June. It was compiled by a Working Group, chaired by Professor Nicholas Day, which was convened by the Director of the PHLS at the request of the Chief Medical Officer. Data were used from the unlinked anonymous HIV prevalence monitoring programme, the National Survey of Sexual Attitudes and Lifestyles[7] and case reports of AIDS. The Group made annual projections up to 1997 of likely numbers of new AIDS diagnoses for the various exposure categories; deaths from AIDS-related diagnoses; people with severe HIV disease who did not meet all the criteria for a diagnosis of AIDS; and total AIDS prevalence. The planning projections are summarised in Table 6.4. Monitoring of the AIDS incidence projections using reports received up to the end of March 1993 has shown that projections published by the same Group in 1990[8] have been accurate (Figure 6.4).

The Working Group estimated that total HIV prevalence in England and Wales at the end of 1991 was approximately 23,400. The Working Group also revised its earlier assessment of the under-reporting of AIDS cases from 20%[9] to 13%. The new report highlighted the differences in the trends between exposure categories

Table 6.4: *Projections of AIDS incidence, mortality, prevalence, and the number of persons with other severe HIV disease (adjusted for under-reporting)*

Year	AIDS			Other severe HIV disease
	New cases (incidence)	Deaths*	Cases alive at year end (prevalence)	Persons alive at year end and requiring care† (prevalence)
1992	1840	1355	3005	3015
1993	2110	1680	3440	3450
1994	2265	1955	3750	3760
1995	2375	2135	3985	3995
1996	2430	2290	4130	4140
1997	2440	2375	4190	4205

*Derived through applying survival life tables to past and future AIDS incidence.
†Prevalent AIDS cases multiplied by 1.003.

Source: *Commun Dis Rep* 1993; **3 (Suppl 1)**

Figure 6.4: *AIDS incidence compared with earlier projections, England and Wales, 1989-93*

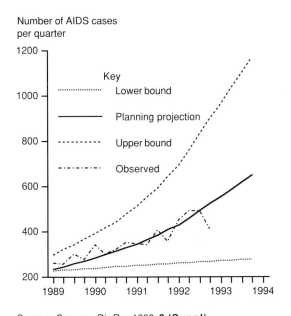

Source: *Commun Dis Rep* 1993; **3 (Suppl)**

Figure 6.5: *Observed (1984-91) and projected (1992-97) annual incidence of AIDS from data to end June 1992, England and Wales*

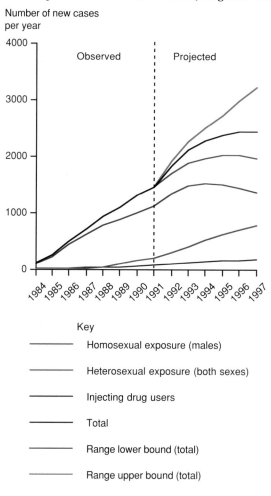

Number of new cases per year

Key

——— Homosexual exposure (males)

——— Heterosexual exposure (both sexes)

——— Injecting drug users

——— Total

——— Range lower bound (total)

——— Range upper bound (total)

Source: *Commun Dis Rep* 1993; **3(Suppl)**

which have been observed and forecast (Figure 6.5). It suggested that AIDS incidence among homosexual men may plateau in 1994 with a slow decline to 1997, but the confidence limits for these projections grow progressively wider from 1993 with the upper range forecast continuing to rise. A steady increase is projected for new AIDS cases among those who have been infected through heterosexual sexual intercourse. The report also suggested that there had been a peak in new HIV infections among injecting drug users in 1985, with a subsequent fall.

It is essential to continue monitoring these projections in view of continued uncertainty about the long-term risks of an epidemic of HIV infection among heterosexual men and women. It will also be important to identify at an early stage any increases in high-risk behaviour among groups already known to be at especial risk of HIV infection.

AIDS/HIV infected health care workers

In 1993, the Department of Health (DH) started to revise guidance on the management of HIV-infected health care workers[10]. An interim document[11] was published for consultation in April and the final guidance will become available in early 1994. The guidance is based on advice and recommendations from the Expert Advisory Group on AIDS and its United Kingdom (UK) Advisory Panel for health care workers infected with bloodborne viruses, and incorporates revised statements on ethical issues from statutory professional bodies.

Guidance[12] was also published in April to advise National Health Service (NHS) managers about notification or 'look-back' exercises for patients treated by an HIV-infected health care worker who have undergone procedures where there may be any risk of HIV transmission. Look-back exercises are appropriate if it is concluded, on the basis of detailed individual consideration of working practices, that the patients should be offered counselling and HIV testing. The UK Advisory Panel of the Expert Advisory Group on AIDS will provide confidential advice as required.

The risk of transmission of HIV infection from health care workers to patients appears to be extremely remote, but is clearly a matter of public concern. DH has set up a Working Group to evaluate this risk; its findings will incorporate a thorough and independent review of all published evidence.

HIV in blood donations

During 1993, 2.92 million blood donations were tested with anti-HIV-1+2 combined tests. Twenty donations (from 16 males and 4 females) were found to be HIV-seropositive, or 1 in 145,942 (0.0007%). The number of new donors tested was 334,000, of whom 11 were seropositive (1 in 30,400, or 0.003%). Again, no donations were found to be anti-HIV-2 positive during 1993.

Table 6.5 shows the number of donations tested in the UK between the autumn of 1985 and the end of 1993, together with the number of donations confirmed as HIV-seropositive. The male:female ratio of seropositive donations in 1993 was 4:1, and among new donors there were 7 male and 4 female seropositive donors. These findings indicate that the 1992 figures probably represent only a temporary change from the previous pattern of most HIV-seropositive blood donations being given by men. As previously, most anti-HIV-seropositive donors were in the age-groups 21-30 and 31-40 years.

Twelve of the 20 donors with HIV infection have been asked about factors that might be relevant to their HIV-seropositivity. Eight of the 10 males who have so far been interviewed had had sex with other men, 1 had another high-risk partner, and 1 was probably infected by heterosexual sexual intercourse. The 2 female donors interviewed probably acquired the infection through heterosexual activity in which the partner could not be readily identified as a member of any high-risk group.

Table 6.5: *HIV in blood donations in the United Kingdom, October 1985 to December 1993*

Year	Donations tested (million)	Donations confirmed HIV-seropositive			
		Male	Female	Total	%
1985	0.6	13	0	13	0.002
1986	2.64	44	9	53	0.002
1987	2.59	18	5	23	0.0009
1988	2.64	18	5	23	0.0009
1989	2.74	25	12	37	0.001
1990	2.82	23*	12	35*	0.001
1991	2.59	23	8	31	0.001
1992	2.90	15	11	26	0.0009
1993	2.92	16	4	20	0.0007
Total	22.80	195	66	261	0.001

*Includes one anti-HIV-2-positive donation.
Minor differences in these figures from those published last year are due to late reporting.

Source: National Blood Authority

Public education and prevention

In January, the Health of the Nation key area handbook on HIV/AIDS and sexual health[13] was published to assist the local development of sexual health education strategies. Regional AIDS control reports for 1992/93 show continued support and development of such work. Many initiatives are innovative and cover wider sexual health issues, but all must be appropriately targeted.

The Health Education Authority (HEA) has continued to run national campaigns on HIV infection and AIDS and sexual health, as well as targeted campaigns for people from ethnic minority groups, and men who have sex with men. In October, an educational video and information booklet[14] for seafarers was launched in association with the British Red Cross and the shipping industry. DH also launched its 'Travel Safe' campaign to alert travellers to the risks of acquiring HIV infection overseas.

In July, DH held a multifaith consultation day, which will lead to a conference in 1994 on HIV/AIDS and Britain's religious communities, organised in conjunction with Oxford Regional Health Authority (RHA).

References

1. Report of a Working Group convened by the Director of the Public Health Laboratory Service on behalf of the Chief Medical Officer. The incidence and prevalence of AIDS and other severe HIV disease in England and Wales for 1992-7: projections using data to the end of June 1992. *Commun Dis Rep* 1993; **3 (Suppl 1)**: S1-S17. Chair: Professor Nicholas Day.
2. Public Health Laboratory Service AIDS Centre. The surveillance of HIV-1 infection and AIDS in England and Wales. *Commun Dis Rep* 1991; **1**: R51-R56.

3.   Waight PA, Rush AM, Miller E. Surveillance of HIV infection by voluntary testing in England. *Commun Dis Rep* 1992; **2**: R85-R90.

4.   Public Health Laboratory Service AIDS Centre at CDSC, PHLS Virus Defence Laboratory, Academic Department of Genito-urinary Medicine University College and Middlesex School of Medicine et al. The unlinked anonymous HIV prevalence monitoring programme in England and Wales: preliminary results. *Commun Dis Rep* 1993; **3**: R1-R11.

5.   Evans BG, Catchpole MA, Heptonstall J et al. Sexually transmitted diseases and HIV-infection among homosexual men in England and Wales. *BMJ* 1993; **306**: 426-8.

6.   Weatherburn P, Hunt AJ, Hickson FCI, Davies PM. *The sexual lifestyles of gay and bisexual men in England and Wales.* London: HMSO, 1992.

7.   Johnson AM, Wadsworth J, Wellings K, Bradshaw S, Field J. Sexual lifestyles and HIV risk. *Nature* 1992; **360**: 410-2.

8.   Report of a Working Group convened by the Director of the Public Health Laboratory Service. Acquired immune deficiency syndrome in England and Wales to end 1993: projections using data to end September 1989. *Commun Dis Rep* 1990 (suppl).

9.   Department of Health, Welsh Office. *Short term prediction of HIV infection and AIDS in England and Wales: report of a working group.* London: HMSO, 1988. Chair: Professor David Cox.

10.   Department of Health. *AIDS-HIV Infected Health Care Workers: occupational guidance for health care workers, their physicians and employers: recommendations of the Expert Advisory Group on AIDS.* Heywood (Lancashire): Department of Health, 1991.

11.   Department of Health. *AIDS-HIV Infected Health Care Workers: guidance on the management of infected health care workers.* Heywood (Lancashire): Department of Health, 1993.

12.   Department of Health. *AIDS-HIV Infected Health Care workers: practical guidance on notifying patients: recommendations of the Expert Advisory Group on AIDS.* Heywood (Lancashire): Department of Health; 1993.

13.   Department of Health. *The Health of the Nation Key Area Handbook: HIV/AIDS and sexual health.* London: Department of Health, 1993.

14.   Health Education Authority. *HIV and AIDS Information for Seafarers.* London: Health Education Authority, 1993.

(b)   Other sexually transmitted diseases

The total number of new cases seen at GUM clinics in England continues to rise, with 656,902 seen in 1992, a rise of 3.5% over 1991 and of 14.7% when compared with 1989 (see Table 6.6); sexually transmitted diseases (STDs) and other infections requiring treatment were diagnosed in just over 55%. Numbers of patients for whom no treatment was required or referral elsewhere was indicated also continued to rise. Overall, the number of reports of confirmed STDs and other infections fell by 2% from 370,524 to 362,940. Of these, approximately 23% were for wart virus infection, 18% for non-specific genital infection, 10% for chlamydia, 7% for herpes simplex virus and 4% for gonorrhoea. All figures are derived from the KC60 reporting form for consultations in NHS GUM clinics. A high proportion of the reports of STDs came from patients in younger age-groups; among women, 70% of post-pubertal uncomplicated gonorrhoea, 70% of post-pubertal uncomplicated chlamydia, 52% of first attacks of herpes simplex and 66% of first attacks of viral warts occurred in those aged under 25 years (see Figure 6.6).

The Health of the Nation initiative set a target to reduce the incidence of gonorrhoea among men and women aged 15-64 years by at least 20% by 1995 (from 61 new cases per 100,000 population in 1990 to no more than 49 new cases per 100,000). In 1992, total reports of gonorrhoea fell by 23.5% compared with 1991, from 18,683 to 14,283, the decrease being roughly equal in men and women (see Figure 6.7); the incidence of gonorrhoea in this age-group fell below the target to 45 cases per 100,000 population. In women just over one-third of cases of post-pubertal uncomplicated gonorrhoea occurred in those under 20 years-of-age, compared with 11.5% among men in this age-group.

Table 6.6: *Sexually transmitted diseases reported by NHS genito-urinary medicine clinics, England, in year ending 31 December 1992*

Condition	Males	Females	Persons
All syphilis	848	464	1312
Infectious syphilis	*228*	*110*	*338*
All gonorrhoea	8744	5539	14283
Post-pubertal uncomplicated	*7961*	*4401*	*12362*
All chlamydia (excluding PID and chlamydial infections with arthritis)[1]	16661	18747	35408
Post-pubertal uncomplicated	*13089*	*15309*	*28398*
Pelvic infection and epididymitis	1338	6437	7775
Non-specific urethritis (NSU) and related disease	48044	16886	64930
Chlamydial infections/NSU with arthritis	330	67	397
Chancroid/Donovanosis/LGV	57	18	75
Trichomoniasis	371	5472	5843
Vaginosis/vaginitis/balanitis	10379	34789	45168
Candidiasis	9104	51618	60722
Scabies/pediculosis	4248	1497	5745
All Herpes simplex	11602	12749	24351
Herpes simplex-first attack	*6140*	*7877*	*14017*
Herpes simplex-recurrence	*5462*	*4872*	*10334*
All Wart virus infections	49450	35150	84600
Wart virus infection-first attack	*27169*	*23955*	*51124*
Wart virus infection-recurrence	*22281*	*11195*	*33476*
Viral hepatitis	528	97	625
Asymptomatic HIV infection - first presentation	1168	255	1423
Asymptomatic HIV infection - subsequent presentation	*8240*	*1102*	*9342*
HIV infection with symptoms, not AIDS - first presentation	1284	149	1433
AIDS - first presentation	1028	96	1124
Other conditions requiring treatment[2]	61230	52645	113875
Other episodes not requiring treatment	94696	80939	175635
Other conditions referred elsewhere	5846	6332	12178
Total new cases seen	326956	329946	656902

[1] Comprises "uncomplicated chlamydial infection", "other complicated chlamydia (excluding PID and epididymitis)" and "chlamydia ophthalmia neonatorum".

[2] Includes epidemiological treatment of trichomoniasis, vaginosis, vaginitis, balanitis and candidiasis.

LGV = lymphogranuloma venereum; PID = pelvic inflammatory disease.

Source: Form KC60

Figure 6.6: *Age distribution of sexually transmitted diseases diagnosed in NHS genito-urinary medicine clinics, England, 1992*

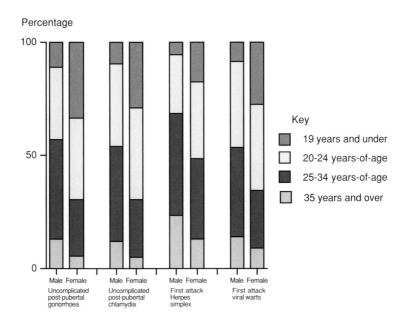

The total number of reports of uncomplicated chlamydia infection fell by 4.2% (1.7% in men and 6.3% in women). Uncomplicated non-specific genital infections fell by 9.3% from 71,575 in 1991 to 64,930 in 1992, this being largely due to an 11% fall in non-specific urethritis among men. There was a further increase of 16.4% in pelvic inflammatory disease among women, from 5,528 in 1991 to 6,437 in 1992; as in previous years, most cases (87%) were not attributable to gonorrhoea or chlamydia.

There was a slight decrease in reports of syphilis, mainly due to a fall in non-infectious syphilis in men. Only 338 cases of infectious syphilis were reported, 10 less than in 1991.

First attacks of herpes simplex virus (HSV) rose in women by 10.6% to 7,877 cases (primarily in the 20-35 years age-group) but were fairly stable in men at 6,140 cases. First attacks of HSV are now more common in women, accounting for 56% of such reports, although men account for 53% of recurrences. Attendances for recurrent attacks of HSV rose by 17% to 5,462 among men and by 25% to 4,872 in women, and accounted for 42% of total reports of HSV. There were slight falls in first attacks of viral warts among men (3.8%) and women (2.0%). However, recurrent attacks increased in men and women and accounted for 40% of all reports of wart virus infection during 1992.

Figure 6.7: *All gonorrhoea: number of new cases seen at NHS genito-urinary medicine clinics, England, 1980-92*

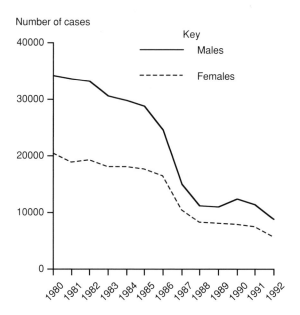

Source: Forms SBH60 and KC60

(c)   Immunisation

Immunisation coverage continues to rise in line with the 1995 targets for childhood vaccination. By September 1993, the 95% uptake targets by the age of 2 years had been reached by 73% of Districts for diphtheria, tetanus and polio vaccines, by 38% for measles, mumps and rubella (MMR) vaccine and by 32% for pertussis vaccine. Despite concerns about shortages of MMR vaccine after altered supply arrangements, national coverage figures were little changed at 92-93%. Since the replacement of MMR vaccines derived from Urabe mumps virus, intensive surveillance has shown no cases of virus-positive mumps meningitis in children recently given MMR vaccine.

In the early part of 1993, there was a rise in notifications and laboratory-confirmed cases of rubella; most of these were among men aged 16-21 years, but there was also an increase in laboratory-confirmed infections among pregnant women (12 in 1991, 2 in 1992, and 25 in 1993). These findings emphasise the need to ensure that all women of child-bearing age are protected against rubella.

Notifications of pertussis, measles and mumps remain at extremely low levels, although there has been an increasing proportion of cases of measles in older age-groups. No cases of indigenous wild virus poliomyelitis were reported.

Haemophilus influenzae *type b*

Immunisation against *Haemophilus influenzae* type b (Hib) was introduced into routine use in October 1992. The programme has been outstandingly successful. Children born in August and September 1992 in South East Thames RHA and Wales who were invited for routine Hib immunisation at 2, 3 and 4 months were subsequently tracked to monitor immunisation uptake. Table 6.7 shows Hib coverage for these children as well as coverage at 12 months-of-age for the first national cohort to be eligible for Hib immunisation.

The national coverage of 92% already equals uptake for pertussis vaccine. One year after its introduction, 37% of Districts reported 95% uptake of Hib vaccination at 12 months.

Table 6.7: *Immunisation coverage for Haemophilus influenzae type b among children born in August/September 1992*

Locality	5 months	8 months	11 months	12 months
SE Thames	53	83	88	90
Wales	71	85	89	93
National	-	-	-	92

Source: PHLS

Figure 6.8: *Reports of Haemophilus influenzae type b infection, 1989-93*

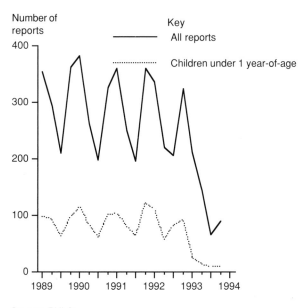

Source: PHLS

155

The impact of immunisation on serious infections caused by Hib has also been dramatic. Figure 6.8 shows the decline in laboratory-confirmed Hib infections (meningitis and septicaemia) reported to PHLS, 1989 to 1993. Invasive Hib disease among all age-groups fell by 63% in 1993 compared with previous years. The fall among children under 1 year-of-age, who are particularly susceptible to Hib, was 85%.

The launch of the Hib immunisation programme was supported by an extensive publicity campaign that included television, newspaper and magazine advertising, aimed particularly at the parents of young children. The impact of this advertising campaign was monitored in studies commissioned by the HEA. Six months after the launch of the campaign, the existence of Hib vaccine was known by 73% of mothers of children under 36 months-of-age and, within that group, by 86% of mothers of children under 12 months-of-age.

(d)   Hepatitis B guidelines

In August, the NHS Management Executive issued new guidelines[1], *Protecting Health Care Workers and Patients from Hepatitis B,* which contained advice from the Advisory Group on Hepatitis. This advice aimed to ensure that health care workers who may be at risk of acquiring hepatitis B virus (HBV) infection from patients are protected by immunisation, and that patients are protected against the risk of acquiring hepatitis B from an infected health care worker. The guidance underlined existing advice that hepatitis B vaccine should be given to all health care workers, including those in training, who are at occupational risk of exposure to HBV.

The guidance also recommends that all health care workers who perform exposure-prone procedures (in which injury to the worker could result in his or her blood contaminating a patient's open tissues) should be immunised against HBV and their response to the vaccine should be checked; health care workers who are highly infectious carriers of hepatitis B (who are HBe-antigen positive) should not carry out such procedures. The guidelines set targets whereby provider units should aim to immunise and check the immunity of all surgeons by the middle of 1994, and of all staff involved in exposure-prone procedures by mid-1995.

Reference

1.   Department of Health. *Protecting Health Care Workers and Patients from Hepatitis B.* Heywood (Lancashire): Department of Health, 1993 (Health Service Guidelines: HSG(93)40).

(e)   Influenza

After a year of very little activity, influenza arrived in the UK earlier than usual during 1993. Unusually, influenza virus was isolated from four sporadic cases during July and August, and the first outbreak, in Scotland, was in early October; thereafter, influenza spread progressively south. General practitioner (GP) consultation rates in England and Wales reached a peak in the second week of

November of 202 per 100,000 population for 'influenza-like illness' and 39 per 100,000 for 'epidemic influenza', comparable to other years of moderate activity. By contrast, rates for 'epidemic influenza' as high as 272 per 100,000 population were recorded during the last influenza epidemic in 1989/90. The Office of Population Censuses and Surveys (OPCS) recorded more deaths from all causes than expected shortly after the peak of new GP consultations, a well-recognised phenomenon, but few deaths were attributed to influenza.

Almost all viral isolates during 1993 were strains of influenza A (subtype H_3N_2), related to the H_3N_2 component of the season's vaccine. In advance of each influenza season, the composition of the influenza vaccine is designed to contain components that are closely related to the virus strain anticipated to be circulating. Vaccine production is matched as far as possible to expected demand, since any unused vaccine is unlikely to be of use in another season, and is produced to tight deadlines after the likely virus strains for the next influenza season have been identified. Extra vaccine supplies may take time to produce and to distribute, and unexpected demand can therefore result in temporary shortages. In 1993, the early onset of the influenza season and increased demand for vaccine because of media speculation about a possible influenza epidemic, combined with delayed availability of vaccine from one manufacturer, led to a temporary shortage, and highlighted some uneven distribution, of vaccine. DH is now reviewing influenza vaccine supply and distribution. Such supply problems would be less likely to occur if doctors could identify those patients most at risk from influenza infection, for whom vaccination is indicated in the memorandum *Immunisation against Infectious Disease*[1] and in advice on influenza vaccination sent out annually by the Chief Medical Officer[2], and order these vaccine supplies well in advance.

References

1. Department of Health. *Memorandum "Immunisation against infectious disease"*. Heywood (Lancashire): Department of Health, 1993 (Professional Letter PL/CMO(92)7).
2. Department of Health. *Influenza immunisation*. Heywood (Lancashire): Department of Health, 1993 (Professional Letter: PL/CMO(93)13).

(f)   Tuberculosis

In April, the World Health Organization (WHO) declared tuberculosis to be a global emergency. Worldwide, WHO estimates that tuberculosis causes 8 million new infections and 3 million deaths annually, mostly in developing countries, but with continued upward trends in Europe and the United States of America (USA). In England and Wales, 5,920 cases were notified in 1993, compared with 5,798 in 1992[1].

The main concerns in Europe and the USA centre on the relation between tuberculosis and the migration of people, HIV infection, and poverty, deprivation and homelessness; the possible emergence of drug resistance; the need to ensure full patient compliance with treatment; and the protection of health care workers.

157

The UK has taken several steps to ensure appropriate policies for the prevention and control of tuberculosis that anticipate likely future trends. DH set up an Inter-Departmental Tuberculosis Working Group to consider which aspects of tuberculosis infection require further action and guidance, and to take these activities forward.

The development of effective policies depends on the availability of appropriate and timely surveillance data. The planned survey of notifications in England and Wales, and a similar survey in Scotland, took place throughout 1993, co-ordinated by the CDSC. The survey included anonymous voluntary HIV testing of tuberculosis patients between the ages of 16 and 54 years. Preliminary results are expected towards the end of 1994. Special surveys of tuberculosis notifications have taken place about every five years since 1965 and have given important information not available from routine notification data, such as the distribution of new cases among ethnic minority groups. However, these surveys have become increasingly subject to delays in obtaining data from hard-pressed clinicians. In June, the PHLS held a workshop to discuss possible future improvements to tuberculosis surveillance, which identified a need for more emphasis on local data collection, with national collation of data for assessment of nationwide trends. Further discussions are under way.

The PHLS also strengthened its monitoring of drug resistance. Between 1982 and 1991, drug-resistant *Mycobacterium tuberculosis* infection remained at a low level in England and Wales[2]. A British Thoracic Society (BTS) Working Group revised the Society's Code of Practice for the prevention and control of tuberculosis. These will be published during 1994, and implementation of guidelines within the wider public health framework will be addressed by the Tuberculosis Working Group during 1994.

The most important measures for the prevention and control of tuberculosis, and for the prevention of drug resistance, are prompt identification of active cases and ensuring that every patient so identified takes a full course of curative chemotherapy. The charity CRISIS again showed that on-site chest radiography was a successful and acceptable method to detect cases of tuberculosis among homeless people who attended its 'Open Christmas' shelter in London. In previous years many patients so identified were later lost to follow-up, but in 1993 closer collaboration with chest physicians enabled quicker investigation and treatment.

References

1. Department of Health. *On the State of the Public Health: the annual report of the Chief Medical Officer of the Department of Health for the year 1992.* London: Department of Health, 1993; 168-9.
2. Warburton ARE, Jenkins PA, Waight PA, Watson JM. Drug resistance in initial isolates of *Mycobacterium tuberculosis* in England and Wales, 1982-1991. *Commun Dis Rep* 1993; **3**: R175-R179.

(g)   Foodborne and waterborne diseases

Foodborne diseases

The number of notifications of food poisoning increased by about 9% in 1993 following a 19% increase in 1992 after three years of reported stability[1]. Compared with 1992, there was little change in the number of laboratory reports received during the year for salmonellosis, campylobacter enteritis and listeriosis, but there was a fall of 18% for isolations of verocytotoxin-producing *Escherichia coli* (VTEC) serogroup 0157, although this organism was isolated for the first time from food (from raw milk and from a beefburger).

Advisory Committee on the Microbiological Safety of Food

The reports of two of the Advisory Committee's first major reviews - of *Salmonella* in eggs[2] and vacuum packaging and associated processes[3] - were published in early 1993. The report on *Salmonella* in eggs[2] endorsed the Government's advice that people should avoid eating raw eggs or uncooked foods made from them and vulnerable groups such as elderly or sick people, babies and pregnant women, should only consume eggs that have been cooked until the white and yolk are solid. The Committee also recommended that eggs should be used within three weeks of being laid and should be stored in a refrigerator after purchase. The report on vacuum packaging and associated processes[3] was produced to ensure that industry, consumers and enforcement authorities are aware of the potential risk of botulism if vacuum or modified atmosphere packaged chilled foods with extended shelf-lives are not produced to the highest standards. The Committee's interim report on *Campylobacter*[4] was published in October. This report reviewed the available information about this micro-organism, identified gaps in knowledge to be addressed and assessed its effects on public health.

The Government has generally accepted these reports' recommendations, many of which have been implemented or are in the process of being implemented. The Committee's first report of progress for 1990-92[5] was also published. Working groups on VTEC 0157 and the poultry meat industry began work in 1993 and made good progress; reports are expected to be submitted to Ministers in 1994. A number of other issues were considered and the Committee made several recommendations for surveillance to the Steering Group on the Microbiological Safety of Food.

Steering Group on the Microbiological Safety of Food

During 1993, the Steering Group continued to develop a microbiological surveillance programme for the food chain. After the completion of a range of pilot studies, major surveys were started on human infectious intestinal disease (IID) in England and the microbiological safety of ready-to-eat meats and meat products. The IID study, which was commissioned from the Medical Research Council (MRC), the London School of Hygiene and Tropical Medicine and the PHLS, will attempt to establish the true incidence of food poisoning, to identify the micro-organisms associated with foodborne disease and risk factors for infection, and to assess the economic costs of IID. More than 20,000 participants will be recruited from 72 general practices throughout England. The study should be completed in 1996 and will cost around £2 million.

Preliminary work on other microbiological food surveillance studies also took place during 1993 and further studies next year should help to assess the microbial contamination of self-service salad bars, the potential sites for contamination in catering premises, and the carriage of VTEC 0l57 in cattle.

The Steering Group's report of progress for 1990-92[6] was published in October; future reports will be published annually.

Notification of food poisoning

The number of cases of food poisoning (formally notified and ascertained by other means) in England and Wales reported to OPCS in 1993 provisionally totalled 69,955. This is an increase of 9% over the 64,336 cases provisionally reported in the first 52 weeks of 1992 (there were 53 reporting weeks for 1992 and the corrected figure for notifications for the whole year was 63,347; see Table 6.8). However, this increase is just under half of that reported between 1991 and 1992.

Salmonellosis

During 1993, the total number of reports of human salmonellosis in England and Wales entered into the PHLS Salmonella Data Set was 30,654, compared with 31,355 for 1992. Isolations of *Salmonella enteritidis* including phage type 4 showed a slight increase but isolation of all other serotypes of *Salmonella* fell. (see Table 6.9). The incidence of *Salmonella typhimurium* definitive type (DT) 104 in human beings almost doubled to just over 1,500 from around 800 in 1992; this increase occurred mainly in the second half of the year, and isolations from

Table 6.8: *Food poisoning: reports to OPCS, England and Wales, 1982-93*

Year	Total*
1982	14253
1983	17735
1984	20702
1985	19242
1986	23948
1987	29331
1988	39713
1989	52557
1990	52145
1991	52543
1992	63347†
1993	69955**

* Statutorily notified to OPCS and ascertained by other means.
† Data for 53 reporting weeks (64,336 [provisional data] for first 52 weeks).
**Provisional data.

Source: OPCS

160

Table 6.9: *Salmonella in human beings, England and Wales, January to December (inclusive) 1992 and 1993*

Serotype	1992		1993**	
	Confirmed isolates	Acquired abroad *(%)*	Confirmed isolates	Acquired abroad *(%)*
S. enteritidis				
Phage type 4	16987	1388 *(8)*	17258	1282 *(7)*
Other phage types	3107	567 *(18)*	2998	498 *(17)*
S. typhimurium	5401	456 *(8)*	4776	445 *(9)*
Others (typed)*	5302	1392 *(26)*	4723	1373 *(29)*
Others (untyped)†	558	101 *(18)*	899	73 *(8)*
All serotypes	31355	3904 *(12)*	30654	3671 *(12)*

*   Salmonellas fully identified as serotypes other than *S. enteritidis* or *S. typhimurium*.
†   Organisms reported without further identification.
** Provisional

Source: PHLS Salmonella Data Set

food animals, mainly cattle, also increased. No single food has been implicated, but the PHLS will maintain particular vigilance on this strain.

Campylobacter enteritis

Campylobacter continues to be the most commonly isolated bacterium associated with acute gastro-enteritis in human beings. The provisional number of laboratory reports to CDSC of faecal isolation of *Campylobacter* in England and Wales during 1993 was 39,385, compared with a revised figure of 38,552 (provisionally reported as 38,556) in 1992.

Listeriosis

Reported cases of listeriosis continue at a low level. There were provisionally 102 reported cases in 1993 compared with a final figure of 106 in 1992.

Verocytotoxin-producing Escherichia coli

The most common VTEC serogroup linked to cases of human illness is 0157. Last year's Report[1] noted that the number of isolations of VTEC 0157 identified by the Laboratory of Enteric Pathogens in England and Wales had increased from one in 1982 to 468 in 1992. During 1993, 390 cases were identified, compared with the revised figure for 1992 of 473. Symptoms range from mild bloody diarrhoea to the haemolytic uraemic syndrome (HUS); isolates associated with HUS are most common among children under 10 years-of-age.

Although most cases are sporadic, a few outbreaks have been reported and in some a foodborne source has now been implicated. Until June 1993, examination of foodstuffs in the UK had failed to detect VTEC 0157 but the organism was then found in raw milk in an outbreak associated with a dairy[7], and was subsequently isolated from a raw beefburger.

The Advisory Committee on the Microbiological Safety of Food is assessing the significance of VTEC as a foodborne pathogen and will advise on any action to be taken to reduce any identified risks from food; the PHLS continues to monitor all VTEC isolations.

Waterborne diseases

The overall quality of public water supplies in England and Wales remains very high[8]. Of the nine outbreaks of cryptosporidiosis reported to CDSC during 1993, drinking water was excluded as a vehicle of infection in five. A case-control study found an association between illness and the consumption of unboiled tap water in one of the outbreaks. Contaminated water from a private supply was thought to be the source of an outbreak in which cases of cryptosporidiosis and *Campylobacter* infection were identified. In none of the waterborne outbreaks were cryptosporidia isolated from the sources of drinking water. No other outbreaks of waterborne infection were reported. During 1993, proceedings of a series of Regional seminars for public health doctors to raise awareness of new water legislation, and of water microbiology in general, were published[9].

References

1. Department of Health. *On the State of the Public Health: the annual report of the Chief Medical Officer of the Department of Health for the year 1992.* London: HMSO, 1993: 174-9.
2. Advisory Committee on the Microbiological Safety of Food. *Report on* Salmonella *in Eggs.* London: HMSO, 1993.
3. Advisory Committee on the Microbiological Safety of Food. *Report on Vacuum Packaging and Associated Processes.* London: HMSO, 1993.
4. Advisory Committee on the Microbiological Safety of Food. *Interim Report on* Campylobacter. London: HMSO, 1993.
5. Advisory Committee on the Microbiological Safety of Food. *Report of progress 1990-1992.* London: HMSO, 1993.
6. Steering Group on the Microbiological Safety of Food. *Report of Progress 1990-1992.* London: HMSO, 1993.
7. Chapman PA, Wright DJ, Higgins R. Untreated milk as a source of verotoxigenic *E. coli* 0157. *Veterinary Record* 1993; **133**: 171-2.
8. Drinking Water Inspectorate, Department of the Environment, Welsh Office. *Drinking Water: a report by the Chief Inspector, Drinking Water Inspectorate, 1992.* London: HMSO, 1993.
9. Department of Health. *Drinking Water Supplies: a microbiological perspective: a series of seminars and workshops for public health physicians and environmental health officers.* London: HMSO, 1993.

(h)   Travel-related disease

Diphtheria in the former Soviet Union

During 1993, it became apparent that the rising number of cases of diphtheria reported from the Russian Federation and the Ukraine over the last few years was continuing and spreading to neighbouring countries. Poland, Finland, Latvia, Lithuania and Norway reported cases epidemiologically linked to the Russian

Federation or the Ukraine. The reasons for this resurgence were complex. The main contributory factor was low immunisation coverage rates in children, but weakened immunity in adults was also a major factor.

The risk to travellers was considered small, but in line with WHO advice the Chief Medical Officer advised all doctors that travellers to the Russian Federation and Ukraine should be immunised against diphtheria[1]. Most people born since 1942 would have received the vaccine in childhood and could be expected to be immune, and a booster dose of vaccine was recommended only for those intending to live or to work with local residents and whose primary immunisation had been given more than 10 years previously. The low-dose vaccine required for adults was in short supply, and as an interim measure doctors were advised to use either a combined tetanus toxoid/low-dose diphtheria vaccine available on a named-patient basis from Merieux UK, or a very small dose (0.1 mL) of the single-antigen diphtheria vaccine for children. Three imported cases of toxigenic diphtheria were reported in 1993, although none were from the former Soviet Union.

Malaria

A total of 1,922 cases of imported malaria in England and Wales were reported to the PHLS Malaria Reference Laboratory during 1993. This was slightly more than the 1,629 cases reported in 1992, but less than the 2,332 cases reported in 1991. Five deaths were attributed to malaria infection. During 1993, new guidelines for prophylaxis against malaria for travellers from the UK were published[2]: these took into account the increased world-wide prevalence of strains of *Plasmodium falciparum* that are resistant to chloroquine, and increased experience of the use of mefloquine as an alternative to chloroquine and proguanil prophylaxis in chloroquine-resistant areas, although important contra-indications to the use of mefloquine were highlighted.

Other infections

Other imported infections reported in 1993 included 151 cases of typhoid fever, 302 cases of hepatitis A and 60 cases of Legionnaire's disease.

References

1. Department of Health. *Diphtheria in the former USSR*. Heywood (Lancashire): Department of Health, 1993 (Professional Letter: PL/CMO(93)9).
2. Bradley D. Prophylaxis against malaria for travellers from the United Kingdom. *BMJ* 1993; **306**: 1247-52.

CHAPTER 7

ENVIRONMENTAL HEALTH AND TOXICOLOGY

(a)   Chemical and physical agents in the environment

(i)   *Small Area Health Statistics Unit*

The establishment and work of the Small Area Health Statistics Unit (SAHSU) has been described in the Reports for 1991[1] and 1992[2]. During 1993, the Unit has continued to investigate cancer incidence and mortality around different types of industrial installation, and a major study of municipal incinerators in the United Kingdom (UK) is nearing completion and should be published during 1994. Also nearing completion are investigations of television and radio transmitters; the Baglan Bay petrochemical works; and producers of vinyl chloride monomer.

Each study requires meticulous analysis and interpretation of the data to decide whether or not the observed rate of cancer is higher than that which may be attributable to chance alone. Data have to be carefully checked for completeness of cancer registration and, as far as possible, allowance has to be made for confounding factors or biases - for example by the use of the Carstairs' index[3] to control for socio-economic influences on health. An important methodological development in 1993 was the installation of a Geographical Information System at SAHSU, which will allow the investigation of shapes other than circles around point sources, and of disease rates in different types of geographical locations, such as coastal areas and along roads. The SAHSU methodology examines the evidence for an increased incidence of disease in a given locality and does not address the issue of causality. If a cluster of disease were to be identified near to an industrial installation, it is likely that further investigations would be necessary to identify possible aetiological factors.

(ii)   *Air pollution episodes*

The Department of Health's (DH's) Advisory Group on the Medical Aspects of Air Pollution Episodes (MAAPE) published its third report, on the oxides of nitrogen, in December[4]. As for the Group's two earlier reports, MAAPE was asked to consider whether advice about personal protective measures during air pollution episodes should be given and, if so, what that advice should be, to whom it should be addressed, and when it should be issued. After a detailed review of published work, the Group concluded that individuals who do not suffer from respiratory disease would be unaffected by the ambient concentrations of nitrogen dioxide that have been recorded in the UK. The Group carefully considered evidence about the effects of nitrogen dioxide upon people with asthma: under laboratory conditions there appeared to be little difference in sensitivity to nitrogen dioxide between people who have asthma and those who do not, but epidemiological evidence indicated that those with asthma may have worse symptoms when ambient concentrations of nitrogen dioxide and associated pollutants are raised. The Advisory Group therefore recommended that advice about air pollution episodes should be made available, especially to people with asthma, whenever ambient concentrations of nitrogen dioxide exceed 300 parts per billion (ppb). This advice is available on a free telephone helpline (0800 556677) and some 250 calls to the number are received daily.

In the UK, episodes of air pollution often involve raised concentrations of more than one pollutant, particularly during winter when concentrations of oxides of nitrogen, sulphur dioxide and airborne particles may all be raised simultaneously. The Advisory Group is now reviewing the need for advice about personal protective measures during air pollution episodes that involve mixtures of pollutants.

At DH's request, the Committee on the Medical Effects of Air Pollutants (COMEAP), chaired by Professor Stephen Holgate, established two subgroups during 1993 - one to advise on possible links between asthma and air pollution, because of concerns about a possible link between changing patterns of air pollution and increased general practitioner (GP) consultations and hospital admissions for asthma, and the second to consider evidence about the possible health effects of airborne particles. COMEAP is expected to produce reports on both these issues by early 1995. The newly formed Medical Research Council (MRC) Institute for Environment and Health, supported by DH and the Department of the Environment, has made research into the health effects of air pollution one of its priorities, and during 1993 the Department of the Environment's Expert Panel on Air Quality Standards started to formulate standards for benzene, ozone, carbon monoxide and 1,3-butadiene which should be published in 1994.

(iii)   Institute for Environment and Health

The creation of an Institute for Environment and Health was proposed in the *Health of the Nation* White Paper[5]. In July, the MRC established such an institute, supported jointly by the Department of the Environment and DH, at its Interdisciplinary Research Centre on Mechanisms of Human Toxicity at the University of Leicester. The Institute for Environment and Health will act as a focus for UK research into the links between environmental quality and health and will also support relevant international programmes. It will complement existing work by Government Departments and agencies such as the Ministry of Agriculture, Fisheries and Food (MAFF) into agricultural matters and food safety, and the Health and Safety Executive into occupational health. One of the first projects involves collaborative research with the World Health Organization (WHO) on the possible health effects of air pollution, in preparation for the second European Conference on Environment and Health to be held in Helsinki in June 1994.

(iv)   NHS response to chemical accidents

Health Service Guidelines issued in August drew attention to the arrangements which should be made by health authorities to plan a response to chemical accidents[6]. Accompanying guidance forms a revised chapter for inclusion in the handbook *Emergency Planning in the NHS: health services arrangements for dealing with major incidents*[7]. District Health Authorities (DHAs) are required to designate an appropriate person to be responsible for access to informed advice on possible risks to the public health, and the preparation of plans to be used in the event of such an incident. Liaison and consultation with other organisations and agencies that would take part in any emergency response is essential to ensure an integrated and effective response to any chemical accident. Specialist toxicology advice which may not be available locally can be obtained from the National Poisons Information Service and, in the case of exceptional incidents, the Chief Medical Officer's Health Advisory Group on Chemical Contamination Incidents.

(v)   Distribution of stable iodine

The use of stable or non-radioactive potassium iodate tablets to block thyroid uptake of radioactive iodine and thus reduce the risk of thyroid cancer in the event of a nuclear accident was widely discussed after the Chernobyl incident in 1986. In the light of recommendations by WHO, and a UK Working Group[8], old stocks of potassium iodate tablets have been replaced with tablets at a new dosage level and in January a letter was sent to all GPs[9] to describe the revised indications for their use, appropriate dosages, contra-indications and relevant administrative details.

In October, DH issued revised guidance about the distribution of these tablets to health authorities[10]. Responsibility for taking the lead in ensuring adequate local plans are made to distribute potassium iodate tablets to members of the public rests with DHAs; responsibility for the physical distribution of these tablets is a matter for local agreement.

References

1. Department of Health. *On the State of Public Health: the annual report of the Chief Medical Officer of the Department of Health for the year 1991*. London: HMSO, 1992: 152.
2. Department of Health. *On the State of Public Health: the annual report of the Chief Medical Officer of the Department of Health for the year 1992*. London: HMSO, 1993: 172.
3. Carstairs V. Deprivation and health in Scotland. *Health Bull (Edinburgh)* 1990; **46**: 162-75.
4. Department of Health. *Oxides of nitrogen: third report of the Advisory Group on the Medical Aspects of Air Pollution Episodes*. London: HMSO, 1993. Chair: Professor Anne Tattersfield.
5. Department of Health. *The Health of the Nation: a strategy for health in England*. London: HMSO, 1992 (Cm. 1986).
6. Department of Health. *Arrangements to deal with health aspects of chemical contamination incidents*. Heywood (Lancashire): Department of Health, 1993 (Health Service Guidelines: HSG(93)38).
7. Department of Health. *Emergency Planning in the NHS: health services arrangements for dealing with major incidents*. London: Department of Health, 1990.
8. Department of Health. *Nuclear Accident Countermeasures: iodine prophylaxis*. London: HMSO, 1991 (Report on Health and Social Subjects no. 39).
9. Department of Health. *Potassium iodate (stable iodine) prophylaxis in the event of a nuclear accident*. Heywood (Lancashire): Department of Health, 1993 (Professional Letter: PL/CMO(93)1).

10. Department of Health. *Nuclear emergency planning in the NHS: distribution of stable iodine (potassium iodate tablets): role of Health Authorities.* Heywood (Lancashire): Department of Health, 1993 (Miscellaneous Circular: 93(50); annex to Health Circular: HC(89)8: addendum).

(b)   Toxicological safety

(i)   *Food chemical hazards*

DH's toxicology and chemical food safety branch, in co-operation with other Government Departments and agencies, NHS poisons units and Consultants in Communicable Disease Control (CsCDC), continually assesses and monitors the toxicological hazards and risks posed by chemical contamination of food. The first priority when any incident is reported is to assess the potential risks to human beings and to ensure that contaminated food does not reach consumers. Accurate toxicological advice must always be available so that, if necessary, appropriate treatment can be started immediately. Reports of incidents are usually made by Environmental Health Officers (EHOs) based at regional offices, by MAFF or directly by food manufacturers. Compliance with toxicological advice issued by the branch is monitored by DH and/or MAFF officials. Details of an emergency telephone advice service on food chemical hazards have been widely distributed within the NHS and to EHOs and local authorities (tel: 071-972 5326).

(ii)   *Food carcinogen prioritisation*

Work continued during 1993 on the development of a scheme to identify and assign relative priorities to chemicals in the food supply that are potentially carcinogenic, so that an objective approach is made to setting priorities, and to ensure concentration of effort on areas of greatest importance to the public health. In outline, each substance dealt with by the scheme is assigned an index according to its carcinogenic hazard to human beings, dietary intake, and the proportion of the population exposed.

These proposals were considered by the Committees on the Carcinogenicity and on the Mutagenicity of Chemicals in Food, Consumer Products and the Environment (COC and COM), which advise on potential mutagenic and carcinogenic hazards. Both Committees supported this pragmatic approach to carcinogen prioritisation if some indication of potency could be included in the hazard assessment, and if attempts could be made to refine exposure estimates, particularly to take account of population subgroups who might be at increased risk. Responses to the second suggestion are being explored with MAFF, which will provide dietary intake data.

In a pilot scheme, COC and COM have been asked to advise on the carcinogenic ranking of polycyclic aromatic hydrocarbons, widespread environmental pollutants often found at low concentrations in many foods. Available data on the mutagenicity and carcinogenicity of these closely related compounds, and various approaches to assess their mutagenic and carcinogenic potency, will be considered.

(iii)   Mineral hydrocarbons in food

During 1993, the Committee on the Toxicity of Chemicals in Food, Consumer Products and the Environment (COT) reviewed the results of new toxicity studies on food additives known as mineral hydrocarbons (MHCs). MHCs are complex mixtures of hydrocarbons and other materials, and may occur as oils or waxes. COT had previously recommended that these additives should not be permitted for use in food. After review of all recent toxicological data, COT re-affirmed its recommendation that mineral hydrocarbons should not be used as food additives, with the exception of two of the waxes tested - for which the Committee set a temporary acceptable daily intake of 0-10 mg/kg body weight. This advice was endorsed by MAFF's Food Advisory Committee.

(iv)   The Advisory Committee on Novel Foods and Processes

The Advisory Committee on Novel Foods and Processes (ACNFP) completed its consideration of a genetically modified brewing yeast during 1993. Data about the yeast's development, selection, use and safety (and of the beer produced) were compared with conventional products. The Committee advised that beer produced by or containing this genetically modified yeast was as safe for human consumption as that produced by conventional yeasts.

ACNFP also advised on herbal preparations produced from the leaves of the creosote bush (*Larrea divaricata*), commonly known as 'chaparral', and concluded that such products should not be sold in the UK[1].

(v)   Pesticides

DH and five other Government Departments participate in schemes to approve and to monitor the use of pesticides in the UK. DH's primary concern is for the safety of the general public, as consumers of food which may contain pesticide residues, and of the users of household and garden pesticides. Although exposure to pesticide residues in food residues is a matter of public concern, the prudent use of pesticides (such as the application of fungicides) can reduce exposure to mycotoxins and lower overall health risks. The Working Party on Pesticide Residues' extensive monitoring of foodstuffs available in the UK, published in 1993[2], showed that most samples contained low or undetectable levels of residues. In the few instances where high residue levels were observed, the risks to public health were considered minimal. However, residues of organochlorine pesticides from environmental contamination found in eels in some parts of the country prompted advice to limit eel consumption in those areas[3].

(vi)   Veterinary drugs and animal feedingstuffs

In response to recommendations made in the report of the Expert Group on Animal Feedingstuffs[4], DH and MAFF reviewed aspects of the control of the safety of animal feedingstuffs which were not covered by existing committees.

Ministers decided that the responsible Departments should regularly review new developments in feed materials, manufacturing processes and feeding practices. Departments should obtain relevant specialist advice on specific issues as necessary.

DH continued to provide advice on human safety aspects of the UK licensing of veterinary drugs by the Veterinary Products Committee (VPC [an independent expert body]), the setting of maximum residue levels for veterinary drugs by the European Community's (EC's) Committee on Veterinary Medicinal Products, and the control of animal feedingstuffs by MAFF.

(vii)   Sheep dips

Sheep dips are insecticidal mixtures used to treat external parasitic diseases of sheep, particularly sheep scab and fly-strike. For many years, sheep dips contained organochlorines but these were abandoned because of concerns about environmental persistence and residues in meat. Since 1985, the vast majority of sheep dips used in the UK have contained organophosphates (OPs) as the active ingredient - in particular propetamphos, diazinon or chlorfenvinphos.

Sheep dips are veterinary medicines licensed under the Medicines Act 1968[5] by MAFF and DH Ministers on advice from the VPC. The licensing system is administered by the Veterinary Medicines Directorate, an agency of MAFF. Dipping of sheep was compulsory until 1992, and many farmers continue to dip their sheep - partly because of continued outbreaks of sheep scab or fly-strike.

The OPs used in sheep dips are cholinesterase inhibitors, which may cause tightening of the chest, constricted pupils, abdominal cramps, muscle tremors and fasciculation, confusion and convulsions. During 1991, farmers dipping sheep complained of various symptoms which they attributed to sheep dips; these could broadly be divided into an acute, transient influenza-like illness or a more varied, longer term group of symptoms that included loss of memory, depression, headache, pyrexia and abnormalities of the peripheral nervous system. Doctors have been advised on topics relating to veterinary drugs and pesticides in 1991[6] and 1993[7]. Research projects are under way to examine the acute toxicity of OP sheep dips, occupational hygiene, the possible neurological effects of OPs in sheep dips and the effects of inhalation of sheep dip aerosol.

The VPC reviewed sheep dips twice during 1993, and decided that existing licences should remain in force but that a Certificate of Competence should be held by people wishing to use OP sheep dips; and that a panel of scientists, reporting to the VPC, should be set up to examine all relevant data and to make recommendations on future research.

References

1.   Advisory Committee on Novel Foods and Processes. *Annual Report for 1993*. London: Department of Health, Ministry of Agriculture Fisheries and Food (in press).

2. Ministry of Agriculture, Fisheries and Food, Health and Safety Executive. *Annual Report of the Working Party on Pesticide Residues: 1992.* London: HMSO, 1993.

3. Ministry of Agriculture, Fisheries and Food. *Eels: advice to consumers.* London: MAFF, 1993 (Food Safety Directorate News Release: FSD 27/93).

4. Ministry of Agriculture, Fisheries and Food. *Report of the Expert Group on Animal Feedingstuffs to the Minister of Agriculture, Fisheries and Food, the Secretary of State for Health and the Secretaries of State for Wales, Scotland and Northern Ireland.* London: HMSO, 1992. Chair: Professor Eric Lamming.

5. *Medicines Act 1968.* London: HMSO, 1968.

6. Department of Health. *Reporting of pesticide incidents.* Heywood (Lancashire): Department of Health, 1991 (Professional Letter: PL/CMO(91)5).

7. Department of Health. *Organophosphorus sheep dips: reducing the risks of exposure.* Heywood (Lancashire): Department of Health, 1993 (Professional Letter: PL/CMO(93)8).

CHAPTER 8

MEDICAL EDUCATION, TRAINING AND STAFFING

(a) Junior doctors' hours

In 1991, the 'New Deal', on junior doctors' hours introduced a plan to reduce them through the use of new working arrangements and explicit limits on contracted hours of duty[1]. Good progress during 1992 enabled the Department of Health (DH) to set a target of 1 April 1993 for the first stage of its implementation, with the aim to eliminate posts contracted for more than a maximum average of 83 hours per week. By 1 April, the number of these posts had fallen to 370, compared with 13,000 recorded in 1990; only 91 such posts remained by 30 September.

Between April 1991 and March 1993, 350 extra consultant and 150 additional staff grade posts were funded to support this initiative, at a cost of £24.5 million in 1992/93. In 1993/94, an extra £12.2 million will be used to establish a further 125 consultant posts and to set up local initiatives.

Regional Task Forces are co-ordinating action to reduce maximum average contracted hours for all junior doctors working on-call in hard-pressed posts to 72 hours per week by 31 December 1994. The number of junior doctors in such posts who were contracted to work for between 73 and 83 hours per week fell from 10,262 in September 1992 to 7,798 in September 1993 - a fall of 24%. Maximum average weekly contracted hours for junior doctors working full or partial shifts should fall to 56 and 64 hours, respectively, by 31 December 1994. Regional Task Forces are encouraging new working patterns, better team working, improved cross-cover, and the redistribution of posts between specialties and sites. In December 1993, the Minister for Health re-affirmed the Government's commitment to the 'New Deal', and announced the release of staff grade posts up to the 10% national ceiling and the freedom for Task Forces, in consultation with postgraduate deans, to vary the numbers of senior house officer (SHO) posts according to local requirements.

Reference

1. Department of Health. *Hours of Work of Doctors in Training: the new deal.* London: Department of Health, 1991 (Executive Letter: EL(91)82).

(b) 'Achieving a Balance'

Achieving a Balance: Plan for Action[1] published in 1987, outlined a package of measures to improve patient care by increasing the proportion of care provided by consultants. The suggested annual expansion in the number of consultant posts of at least 2% has been exceeded, and averaged 3.0% annually from 1987 to 1992 when the effects of centrally funded initiatives, including those to reduce junior doctors' hours, are taken into account.

The Joint Planning Advisory Committee (JPAC) continued its regular scrutiny of registrar and senior registrar numbers during the year. In December, a Working Party established by JPAC to consider academic and research quotas produced its report on numbering trainees, programmes and posts which will be published early in 1994. JPAC accepted this report and its recommendations will support the implementation of the recommendations of the report of the Working Group on Specialist Medical Training[2].

In June, the Minister for Health commissioned a review of the achievability of medical staffing policies, and in a response to this report in December he emphasised the Government's commitment to achieving the 'New Deal' targets and announced changes to the planning mechanisms to achieve these targets[3].

References

1. Newton T, Grabham AH, Roberts G. *Hospital Medical Staffing: Achieving a Balance: plan for action: a report issued by the steering group for implementation on behalf of the Health Department, the Joint Consultants Committee and the Chairmen of Regional Health Authorities.* London: Department of Health and Social Security, 1987.
2. Department of Health. *Hospital Doctors: training for the future: the report of the working group on specialist medical training.* London: Department of Health, 1993. Chair: Dr Kenneth Calman.
3. Department of Health. *Minister endorses measures to tackle shortfall of doctors in 21st century.* London: Department of Health, 1993 (Press Release H93/710).

(c)   Medical Manpower Standing Advisory Committee

In April, the Secretary of State for Health accepted the recommendations of the first report of the Medical Manpower Standing Advisory Committee (MMSAC)[1]. Progress has been made towards each of the Committee's recommendations. United Kingdom (UK) medical school student intake in 1993 met the new target of 4,470 and opportunities for flexible working and training were extended. Research was commissioned into the costs associated with increases to the medical workforce and the pattern of doctors' careers. MMSAC continues to consider key issues that might affect the future supply of and demand for doctors and its next report is expected by the end of 1994.

Reference

1. Department of Health. *Planning the Medical Workforce: Medical Manpower Standing Advisory Committee: first report.* London: Department of Health, 1993.

(d)   Equal opportunities for doctors

Equality of opportunity in employment remains a major priority within the National Health Service (NHS). Several policies to improve the conditions for all doctors who are considering a career as a hospital specialist will particularly benefit women. The 'New Deal' initiative on junior doctors' hours[1] and the recommendations of the Working Party on Specialist Medical Training[2] will introduce focused, structured training, usually based in one geographical area, with a defined end-point (the Certificate of Completion of Specialist Training [CCST]). Trainees will have a reasonable expectation of appointment to a consultant post in their early thirties, so that lifestyle and family commitments can be planned in advance.

The report of the Joint Working Party on Flexible Training, issued in April[3], recommended that appointments procedures for the senior registrar flexible training scheme should be devolved to Regional Health Authorities (RHAs) where possible. The new arrangements came into effect from 1 August 1993, and the guidance on flexible training was updated to include information on the new arrangements as well as useful addresses for additional sources of careers guidance. 574 senior registrar posts have been approved for flexible training, 395 of which were filled in December 1993. For registrars, the flexible training scheme will be financed centrally for 1993/94, after which funding will be included in RHAs' baseline allocations. By 31 March 1994, 290 career registrars' posts should be funded under this scheme, an increase of more than 90 since the beginning of 1993, at a cost of over £3 million.

The second Women in Surgical Training (WIST) conference in May was addressed by Baroness Cumberlege, Parliamentary Under Secretary of State in the House of Lords, and was attended by over 150 delegates, many of whom were in SHO or registrar posts[4]. In October, DH organised a conference to allow medical Royal Colleges, RHAs and postgraduate deans the opportunity to share ideas and information on equal opportunities practice, and several ideas from this are under review. Regular monitoring of consultant medical appointments by race and gender has been instituted.

In December, the Secretary of State for Health announced a new initiative on equal opportunities for NHS employees from ethnic minorities[5]. For doctors, it aims to ensure that career and senior registrars from ethnic minorities spend no longer in higher specialist training than caucasian doctors, and to improve the monitoring of their career progress.

References

1. Department of Health. *Hours of Work of Doctors in Training: the new deal.* London: Department of Health, 1991 (Executive Letter: EL(91)82).
2. Department of Health. *Hospital Doctors: training for the future: the report of the Working Group on Specialist Medical Training.* London: Department of Health, 1993. Chair: Dr Kenneth Calman.
3. Department of Health. *Flexible Training: report of the joint working party on flexible training.* London: Department of Health, 1993.
4. Royal College of Surgeons of England. *Women in Surgical Training Schemes.* London: Royal College of Surgeons, 1993.
5. Department of Health. *Ethnic Minority Staff in the NHS: a programme of action.* Leeds: Department of Health, 1993.

(e)   Part-time consultant scheme

The part-time consultant scheme, announced in April 1993[1], provides pump-priming central funding to stimulate the creation of new, part-time consultant posts so that the NHS does not lose the skills of highly trained medical staff whose individual circumstances prevent them from taking up a full-time appointment. This scheme will include senior registrars who have successfully completed part-time training.

Over 500 bids from employing bodies were carefully assessed and 85 new posts, spread across the whole range of medical specialties and across RHAs, were approved in September; the first of the new part-time consultants took up their posts towards the end of the year. Central funding for the posts will continue until March 1996, after which funding should be secured through purchaser contracts in the normal way. It is expected that a second round of bids will be invited in the Spring of 1994.

Reference

1. Department of Health. *Medical and Dental Staffing: part time consultants.* Heywood (Lancashire): Department of Health, 1993 (Executive Letter: EL(93)39).

(f)   New career structure for doctors in community health

Work on the establishment of a new career structure for doctors in child health, including arrangements to assimilate senior clinical and clinical medical officer grades into the mainstream hospital staffing structure as part of a combined child health service, continued during 1993. Formal negotiations with the medical profession were completed by the end of 1993 and guidance should be issued in 1994. Other specialties will be reviewed when the impact of changes in the child health services has been assessed.

(g)   Postgraduate, continuing and specialist medical education

In December, the Minister for Health announced[1] that the Government had accepted in full the recommendations in the Working Group Report on Specialist Medical Training[2]. The measures outlined will comply with European Community legislation, and include shorter, better structured and more intensive programmes of training; the introduction of the CCST, to be awarded by the General Medical Council (GMC) on the recommendation of the medical Royal Colleges; and the introduction of a unified higher training grade to replace existing registrar and senior registrar posts. Implementation of these measures will depend on the capacity of the NHS to assimilate the changes within existing budgets. Further work on the implications of the report for the training of general practitioners, overseas doctors and those following a career in academic and research medicine will be carried out during 1994.

Interim arrangements for the funding of medical and dental training grade posts were introduced from 1 April, when postgraduate deans became responsible for the payment of 50% of basic salary costs and 100% of non-salary costs for all medical and dental trainees. Early reports indicate that this initiative has helped to safeguard training posts, raised the profile of medical and dental training and education and helped to even out training costs. The Joint Working Group on the Funding of Medical and Dental Training Grade Posts is due to make recommendations for long-term arrangements to complement the measures announced in the Calman Report[2], in the Summer of 1994.

As part of a strategy to create a more effective and flexible structure for general practitioner (GP) postgraduate education, GP clinical tutors were brought into the postgraduate deans' education network and on 1 April became eligible for sessional payments as RHA employees, able to work interchangeably with GP course organisers.

During 1993, a need to co-ordinate the various approaches to continuing education by the medical Royal Colleges and others, and to devise a national, affordable strategy, became apparent. In December, a workshop on continuing medical education in Leeds enabled invited participants to exchange ideas, and a consultative document will be launched at a national conference in the Summer of 1994.

References

1. Department of Health. *Minister endorses measures to tackle shortfall of doctors in 21st century.* London: Department of Health, 1993 (Press Release: H93/710).
2. Department of Health. *Hospital Doctors: training for the future: the report of the Working Group on Specialist Medical Training.* London: Department of Health, 1993. Chair: Dr Kenneth Calman.

(h)   Undergraduate medical and dental education

During 1993, the Steering Group on Undergraduate Medical and Dental Education and Research - which monitors the effects of the NHS reforms on, and considers the arrangements for, teaching and research - published its third report[1]. The report, which was endorsed by the Secretaries of State for Health and for Education, emphasised the continued need for joint working between the NHS and universities. It recommended that RHAs should agree contracts for the Service Increment for Teaching and Research (SIFTR) with universities, rather than rely on consultation alone, and identified topics that required continued monitoring or further work, such as the funding of dental hospitals and the service support costs of academic general practice. The Group's terms of reference have now been expanded to allow consideration of the national implications of changes caused by implementation of *Making London Better*[2], and changes to the pre-registration house officer year and the undergraduate medical curriculum.

A scheme was started in 1993 to help English medical schools to introduce changes to undergraduate medical education proposed by the GMC. £1 million were made available to be used, in part, to fund a facilitator at each medical school who would assist the progress of required change, and a further £200,000 were provided to help to develop the dental curriculum, with particular emphasis on exploring common teaching between dentistry and medicine. During the year, university departments of general practice received £468,000, their fourth payment from a fund set up in 1990.

References

1. Department of Health. *Undergraduate Medical and Dental Education Research: third (interim) report of the Steering Group.* Heywood (Lancashire): Department of Health, 1993.
2. Department of Health. *Making London Better.* Heywood (Lancashire): Department of Health, 1993.

(i)   Doctors' performance

In September, the Secretary of State for Health set up a Review Group to assess guidance in relation to the performance of doctors, with terms of reference "To review current guidance and procedures relating to doctors whose performance appears to fall below acceptable standards", and "to make recommendations (by 31 December 1993) to the Secretary of State for any necessary changes and further work necessary".

Early discussions identified a wide range of issues for further consideration including behaviour, communication, attitudes of doctors to patients and education. The Review Group also considered it essential to hear the views of a broad range of representative bodies. Despite considerable progress, the extent of the work identified meant that the Group could not meet its original deadline but will continue its work programme and report by the end of 1994. Oral evidence will be taken early in 1994 from a wide range of groups representing professional, patient and NHS interests as well as the independent sector.

The Review Group's remit does not include the GMC's proposals for new performance procedures or its role as the regulatory body for doctors, and is independent of work on NHS complaints procedures. The overriding aim of the review is to ensure that all patients, whether in the NHS or the private sector, are treated by doctors whose professional skills and competence are satisfactory and safe.

(j)   Locum doctors

A Working Group was set up in December to examine ways to improve quality control in relation to locum doctors who work in the NHS and to ensure that high professional standards are maintained; it is expected to report in the Summer of 1994. Existing guidelines for employers generally seem to work well but occasional problems with unsatisfactory locum doctors have occurred. The Working Group will assess the causes of such difficulties, and make recommendations to minimise any risk to standards of patient care. The Working Group includes representatives from the GMC, medical professional bodies, NHS management, locum agencies and the UK Health Departments.

CHAPTER 9

OTHER TOPICS OF INTEREST IN 1993

(a)   Medicines Control Agency

(i)   *Role and performance*

The Medicines Control Agency (MCA) is an executive agency that reports through its Chief Executive to the Secretary of State for Health. Its role is to advise Ministers and to protect the public health through the control of human medicines, and its primary concern is that medicines available to the public should meet the most stringent criteria for safety, efficacy and quality.

On behalf of Health Ministers (the Licensing Authority), the MCA approves medicines for marketing through the provision of a licence, monitors medicines after licensing, takes action to resolve drug safety concerns and carries out inspection and enforcement under the provisions of the Medicines Act 1968[1], associated United Kingdom (UK) legislation and the relevant European Community (EC) Directives. The MCA also supports the work of the British Pharmacopoeia Commission in setting quality standards for drug substances. The MCA is financed by fees charged to the pharmaceutical industry but aims to set fees no higher than necessary, and continuously reviews the quality of its service. The Agency achieved Trading Fund status in April.

The MCA is responsible for medicines control policy within the Department of Health (DH) and represents the UK in pharmaceutical regulation within the EC and other international settings. During 1993, the MCA has met most of its key targets for licensing despite a further increase in product licence applications and variations, including a 100% increase of simple abridged applications compared with 1992. It continues to be a major rapporteur in the EC Multi-State and concertation procedures. Pharmocovigilance initiatives included the introduction of periodic safety updates from companies for new medicines and new guidances on post-marketing surveillance. Procedures and guidelines for moving medicines from Prescription Only (POM) to Pharmacy (P) status were streamlined, and legislation was introduced in respect of leaflets and labels for medicinal products, homoeopathic medicines, and the wholesale distribution of human medicinal products. The first gene therapy clinical trial was assessed and draft guidance issued. The 1993 edition of the British Pharmacopoeia[2] and information about the work of the agency[3,4,5] were published during the year.

(ii)   *Control of UK clinical trials*

Patients in clinical trials are protected by a system of authorisations and monitoring procedures laid down by legislation[1,6,7,8] and incorporated in guidance notes for applicants who sponsor such trials. In 1993, the MCA approved about 250 new applications for Clinical Trial Exemptions (CTXs), dealt with 2,500 notifications of change to CTXs, and monitored reports of over 3,500 adverse drug events.

The procedures for authorising clinical trials were reviewed as part of the Government's deregulation initiative to ease the administrative burden on industry and to increase the resources available for key objectives. As a result, suggestions to ease the current very strict requirements for notifying any change made to a clinical trial were proposed, and guidance notes on applications for clinical trials were rewritten to simplify the application procedure and to ease some requirements for pre-clinical studies. In addition, the introduction of a Usage Guideline was proposed; such guidelines would specify conditions within which changes to a clinical trial could be set up without informing the Licensing Authority. Consultation on these proposals, which will not compromise the safety of subjects, started during 1993 with a view to legislation during 1994. The MCA also installed a new computer database to improve the handling of applications for clinical trials and the monitoring of their progress. This database stores summaries of information from each clinical trial application and from adverse drug reaction reports.

(iii)   *Reclassification of medicines from Prescription Only to Pharmacy status*

In January, the MCA introduced a new structured annual timetable for changes to the POM Order[9] to expedite the reclassification of POM medicines so that they may be sold over-the-counter from pharmacies. Safety remains the criterion to determine whether or not a medicine can move from prescription control. These procedural changes do not affect the requirement under the Medicines Act 1968[1] for Ministers to consult representative organisations and take account of the advice of the Medicines Act advisory committees before amendments are made to the POM Order. The first amending Order[10] under new arrangements changed 12 medicines from POM to P status, including two histamine-2-receptor blockers (cimetidine and famotidine) at low doses for treating dyspepsia.

(iv)   *Control of gene therapy products*

The quality, safety and efficacy of genetic material for therapeutic use are covered by the Medicines Act[1] and relevant EC Directives, and are therefore the responsibility of the Licensing Authority served by the MCA. In this new and rapidly developing area of research, the MCA works closely with the Gene Therapy Advisory Committee (GTAC), which advises Ministers on whether clinical research proposals are acceptable on ethical grounds; the Advisory Committee on Genetic Modification, which advises the Health and Safety Executive (HSE) and other Government Departments on the human health and safety aspects of work that involves genetic modification; and the Advisory Committee on Releases into the Environment, which advises the Department of the Environment, the HSE and other Government Departments on the risks of deliberate release of genetically modified organisms into the environment.

The first clinical trials were approved during 1993 (see page 185). Guidelines on applications for clinical trials and the production of gene therapy products are being prepared by the MCA and working parties of the Committee for Proprietary Medicinal Products (CPMP). From January 1995, gene therapy products will be subject to the European Medicines Evaluation Agency's (EMEA's) centralised procedure of licensing.

(v)   ***Other pharmaceutical developments in the European Community***

The MCA completed the implementation of EC Directives to harmonise Member States' rules for wholesale distribution of medicines for human use (92/25/EEC) and to set out detailed requirements for applications for product licences (91/507/EEC, amending the Annex to 75/318/EEC). Work to implement Directives on Advertising (92/28/EEC) and Homoeopathic products (93/73/EEC) drew nearer to completion.

During 1993, most EC activity centred on preparation for the introduction of the Future Systems for licensing and pharmacovigilance of pharmaceutical products (see page 197). The MCA took part in conferences of assessors, the development of new guidelines and procedures for all aspects of licensing and pharmacovigilance, and continued its role as a major rapporteur. The MCA has taken a lead in setting standards for information networks within the EC, to form the basis for the transmission of licensing and pharmacovigilance information to all relevant parties.

References

1. *The Medicines Act 1968*. London: HMSO, 1968.
2. Medicines Commission. *British Pharmacopoeia 1993*. London: HMSO, 1993.
3. Medicines Control Agency. *Towards Safe Medicines*. London: HMSO, 1993.
4. Medicines Control Agency. *Rules and Guidance for Pharmaceutical Manufacturers 1993*. London: HMSO, 1993.
5. Medicines Control Agency. *Working with Business: a code of practice*. London: MCA, 1993.
6. Department of Health. *On the State of the Public Health: the annual report of the Chief Medical Officer of the Department of Health for the year 1991*. London: HMSO, 1992; 149.
7. *The Medicines (Exemption from Licences) (Special Cases and Miscellaneous Provisions) Order* 1972. London: HMSO, 1972.
8. *The Medicines (Exemption from Licences) (Clinical Trials) Order* 1981. London: HMSO, 1981.
9. *The Medicines (Products Other Than Veterinary Drugs) (Prescription Only) Order 1983*. London: HMSO, 1983 (Statutory Instrument: SI 1983 no. 1212).
10. *The Medicines (Products Other than Veterinary Drugs) (Prescription Only) Amendment (no. 2) Order 1993*. London: HMSO, 1993 (Statutory Instrument: SI 1993 no. 3256).

(b)   The European Medicines Evaluation Agency and pharmaceutical licensing systems

In June and July, the EC's Internal Market Council adopted a Regulation and three Directives setting out the legal framework of the EC's new medicines licensing arrangements (Future Systems). From 1 January 1995, two new EC licensing procedures will be introduced: a centralised procedure for certain high-technology medicines, which will lead to the grant of a single licence valid across the EC, and a decentralised procedure for other medicines, based on mutual recognition of national licensing decisions, with binding arbitration in the event of disagreement between Member States. Community licensing decisions on medicines for human use will be based on opinions delivered by the EC's CPMP, and the EMEA will provide administrative support for the new procedures and help to co-ordinate post-licensing controls. In October, EC Heads of Government agreed that the EMEA should be based in London.

The principles underlying the Future Systems will ensure the highest standards of assessment work and scientific credibility, and make maximum use of the expertise of national licensing authorities. Member states will be mainly responsible for all post-licensing controls, including pharmacovigilance and inspection, with the EMEA having a role in co-ordination and arbitration in these areas. In the Autumn, work began to draw up a range of EC guidelines, based on these principles, to govern the operation of the new procedures. The EC also circulated for discussion draft Regulations proposing fees to be levied on the pharmaceutical industry by the EMEA for work under centralised and national licensing procedures. Negotiations continued on the development of new arrangements to deal with variations in practice between Member States. Work also started on amendments to bring UK law into line with the Future Systems legislation and to prepare the MCA to operate under these new arrangements.

(c) National Blood Authority

The National Blood Authority (NBA) was set up on 1 April with the responsibility for strategic planning and management of blood services in England to enhance their quality and cost efficiency. The NBA took over the roles of the Central Blood Laboratories Authority, which managed the Bio-Products Laboratory and the International Blood Group Reference Laboratory, and the National Directorate of the National Blood Transfusion Service (NBTS). In April 1994, the NBA will also take over responsibility for the Regional Transfusion Centres.

One of the activities of the National Directorate of the NBTS was to collate figures for blood donors found to be HIV positive (see page 149) or to have evidence of antibodies to hepatitis C virus (HCV). In 1993, 0.33% of donations were HCV-positive on initial screening for hepatitis C, compared with 0.4% in 1992; 0.16% were repeatedly positive, compared with 0.26% in 1992. Supplementary testing confirmed 486 donations (0.017% overall) to be positive, compared with 0.03% in 1992; the number of donations that gave an indeterminate result also fell.

(d) Creutzfeldt-Jakob disease surveillance

A report from Australia indicated a possible link between the occurrence of Creutzfeldt-Jakob disease (CJD), a progressive and fatal neurological disorder, and parenteral treatment with human pituitary gonadotrophins derived from the pituitary glands of cadavers[1]; 4 of some 1,500 women so treated in Australia

Table 9.1: *Creutzfeldt-Jakob disease (CJD) and Gerstmann-Straussler-Scheinker syndrome (GSS), United Kingdom, 1985-93*

Year	Creutzfeldt-Jakob disease			GSS	Total	Sporadic incidence/ million population*
	Sporadic	Iatrogenic	Familial			
1985	26	1	1	0	28	0.49
1986	26	0	0	0	26	0.46
1987	23	0	0	1	24	0.42
1988	21	1	1	0	23	0.40
1989	28	1	1	0	30	0.53
1990	26	5	0	0	31	0.54
1991	32	1	3	0	36	0.63
1992	44	2	4	1	51	0.89
1993	34	3	1	1	39	0.70

*Based on UK population of 57.07 million (1988 Census Update).

Note: These figures may differ from those published previously because the Unit is still identifying cases from previous years.

Source: UK CJD Surveillance Unit

have now been found to have evidence of CJD. About 300 women received similar treatment at a small number of hospitals in the UK between 1956 and 1985. The Government decided that these women should be traced and offered counselling: an advice centre was set up at the Jessop Hospital for Women, Sheffield, under the supervision of Professor Ian Cooke, and its role was described by the Chief Medical Officer in August[2].

Public anxiety about CJD continued throughout the year with considerable media coverage. The incidence of the disease in the UK rose from 0.49 per million population (26 patients) in 1985 to 0.89 per million population (44 patients) in 1992, but fell to 0.7 per million population (34 patients) in 1993 (see Table 9.1). The small increase noted in the 1990s may result from improved ascertainment of cases by the National CJD Surveillance Unit, based in Edinburgh, which was set up in 1990. The annual incidence of CJD in the UK reflects the worldwide distribution, which is 0.5-1 per million population[3]. There remains no scientific evidence for any link between CJD in man and bovine spongiform encephalopathy (BSE) in cattle.

References

1. Cochius JI, Mack K, Burns RJ, Alderman CP, Blumbergs PC. Creutzfeldt-Jakob disease in a recipient of human pituitary-derived gonadotrophin. *Aust NZ J Med* 1990; **20**: 592-3.
2. Department of Health. *Creutzfeldt-Jakob disease from treatment with human pituitary gonadotrophin.* Heywood (Lancashire): Department of Health, 1993 (Professional Letter: PL/CMO(93)11).
3. Brown P, Cathala F, Raubertas RF, Gajdusek DC, Cataigne P. The epidemiology of Creutzfeldt-Jakob disease: conclusion of a 15-year investigation in France and review of the world literature. *Neurology* 1987; **37**: 895-904.

(e)   Medical devices

Medical devices provide the technology which assists and permits the practice of medicine. There is a wide range, from relatively simple devices, such as sutures, syringes and needles, to feedback control systems in intensive care units. The Medical Devices Directorate (MDD) was established in August 1990 to safeguard public health by ensuring that such devices meet appropriate standards of safety, quality and performance.

National retrieving and investigation centre

During 1993, MDD received over 2,700 reports of adverse incidents related to medical devices, of which some 2,000 came from users in UK health services. After initial assessments half of these reports were investigated in depth, the others being subject to a simpler review. As a result of these investigations, MDD issued 12 Hazard Notices and 40 Safety Action Bulletins, as well as other device-related advice.

European Medical Devices Directives

Three EC Directives regulating the safety and marketing of medical devices will come into effect over the next few years, and will eventually replace existing systems in Member States. The UK has played an active part in these initiatives and negotiations to bring about a single European market in medical devices.

Active Implantable Medical Devices Directive

The Active Implantable Medical Devices Directive[1] came into force on 1 January 1993. During a two-year transition period, manufacturers of active implantable medical devices may choose to follow existing national systems of control or the provisions of this Directive. Thereafter all devices for the EC market will need to be approved by an independent certification organisation, the Notified Body for CE Marking.

Under the provisions of this Directive, the Competent Authority received 11 applications for clinical trials of medical devices: 5 were rejected; no objections were raised for 4; and the other 2 are under consideration. Reasons for rejection included statistical, technical and sterilisation problems and unnecessarily high clinical trial populations. Rejected proposals may be resubmitted once the problems have been addressed, and those considered so far have been approved. The Competent Authority has received 2 reports of adverse incidents under the Vigilance System. One Notified Body has been accredited and another application is close to accreditation. A cost compliance assessment of the regulations is close to completion.

Medical Devices Directive

The Medical Devices Directive was adopted by the Internal Market Council in June 1993. It will come into effect in the UK and other Member States on 1 January 1995, with a transitional period to June 1998 during which manufacturers may choose to follow existing national controls, such as the Manufacturer Registration Scheme, or the provisions of the Directive. From 14 June 1998, all except in-vitro diagnostic medical devices marketed through the EC will have to bear the 'CE mark'. Work has started on implementation of this Directive in the UK so that Notified Bodies can be accredited in good time.

In-vitro Diagnostic Medical Devices Directive

A formal proposal from the European Commission for a Directive on in-vitro diagnostic medical devices is likely to be published during 1994 and will then be discussed in the Council of Ministers' Working Group before submission to the Council of Ministers and the European Parliament.

Clinical investigation under the Medical Devices Directives

Devices within high-risk categories or that incorporate novel features or new materials coming into contact with the human body will need clinical data to show that they conform with the Essential Requirements of EC Directives. Such clinical data should take account of the possible adverse effects and potential benefits of the use of the device, and long-term experience with established alternatives, if relevant. From January 1993, manufacturers of active implantable medical devices have to inform the Competent Authority at least 60 days before the clinical investigation of such a device is due to begin, and submit all necessary documents for assessment by relevant officials and external assessors with an expert knowledge of the device or relevant aspects such as sterilisation, materials or toxicology. Manufacturers will be notified if any objections have been raised to the investigation proceeding and will be fully informed of the grounds for any objection, and are free to resubmit the application if the original reasons for the objection have been addressed. All proposals for clinical investigation must also be referred to the relevant Local Research Ethics Committee (LREC), although the Competent Authority can prohibit an investigation on the grounds of public safety even if an LREC has approved the investigation.

Foetal monitoring

Cardiotocography, the continuous electronic monitoring of the foetal heart rate and uterine pressure, has been used to determine foetal health during labour for over 20 years. However, its reliability has been questioned and alternative techniques are under review. In January, the MDD sponsored a conference on foetal monitoring. New methods to record foetal electrocardiograms may prove more sensitive and reliable, but it is essential to ensure that any new monitoring techniques are rigorously evaluated before coming into general use. Studies in this area continue at DH's evaluation unit in Nottingham.

Reference

1. *Active Implantable Medical Devices Regulations 1992.* London: HMSO, 1992 (Statutory Instrument: SI 1992 no. 3146).

(f)   Bioethics

(i)   *Local Research Ethics Committees*

DH Guidelines issued in August 1991 required each District Health Authority (DHA) to establish an LREC to advise on the ethical acceptability of research proposals involving human subjects. These Guidelines were widely welcomed but are kept under continual review. During 1993, DH consulted widely on appropriate training for members of LRECs and ways to streamline procedures to ease the process of ethics committee approval for multicentre research across a large number of health Districts; the responses are now being evaluated. Encouragingly, Regional Directors of Research and Development (RDsRD) have shown considerable interest in LREC training programmes.

(ii)   *Bioethics in Europe*

The Council of Europe's Steering Committee on Bioethics (CDBI) is charged by the Committee of Ministers to study the impact of progress in biomedical sciences on law, ethics, and human rights. The working party of CDBI chaired by Dr Michael Abrams, formerly Deputy Chief Medical Officer, continued to develop proposals for a framework bioethics convention; a draft version should be published during 1994. Three protocols - on organ transplantation, medical research, and the protection of the human embryo and the foetus - are planned under this convention.

During 1993, CDBI organised a symposium on the theme of 'ethics and human genetics'. The UK was strongly represented at this successful and well attended event.

(iii) Committee on the Ethics of Gene Therapy

The report of the Committee on the Ethics of Gene Therapy chaired by Sir Cecil Clothier, whose work was described in the Report for 1991[1], was published in 1992[2]. The Committee emphasised that before gene therapy is introduced into medical practice it must be ethically acceptable and shown to be safe. There were four other main recommendations:

- gene therapy raises no new ethical issues, but because such treatments are so new they should be regarded as research and therefore subject to existing ethical codes for research involving patients;

- gene therapy should be restricted to the alleviation of disease in individual patients, and not used to change or to enhance any normal human characteristics;

- gene modification of sperm or ova, or the cells that produce them, should not at present be attempted because there is insufficient knowledge to evaluate the risk to future generations; *and*

- a non-statutory, expert supervisory body should be set up to work in conjunction with local research ethics committees to assess proposals for gene therapy research.

Following wide consultation, Ministers accepted the recommendations of the Committee and announced the establishment of a new non-statutory body, the Gene Therapy Advisory Committee (GTAC)[3] (see page 136).

The CEGT was asked to remain in being to consider any proposals that might be made to conduct gene therapy research on human subjects before substantive arrangements were in place. As constituted, the Committee did not have the range and depth of very specialised expertise needed to make a wholly satisfactory assessment of all proposals that might be made to conduct gene therapy, particularly in relation to their safety and likely efficacy. The Committee was therefore strengthened by the establishment of an external advisory group whose members acted as expert referees. As gene therapy research increased, the membership of this advisory group was extended to include all necessary expertise. During 1993, under the transitional arrangements operated by the Committee, the first three gene therapy research trials in the UK received ethical approval.

(iv)   Ethics of genetic screening

Increased knowledge of genetics and the mapping of the human genome makes it possible, with varying degrees of precision, to identify specific dispositions and susceptibilities to disease in individuals and their relatives. At present, except in a minority of instances, the predictive power of genetic information is unsure or imprecise. Nevertheless, the prospect of the availability of genetic screening programmes for an increasing number of disorders has caused concern and debate about consent, confidentiality, and the possible implications for employment, health and life insurance, and public policy. These issues must be addressed before any screening programme can be implemented.

During 1992, a letter to Regional General Managers[4] from the National Health Service (NHS) Management Executive included genetic services among services which needed to be kept under review. To assist managers in that review, the Chief Medical and Nursing Officers drew attention to a guide, *Population Needs and Genetic Services*[5], which had been prepared for colleagues who were not specialists in the field. This letter was widely distributed and included guidance on the factors to be taken into account in genetic screening.

The Nuffield Council on Bioethics established a Working Party to consider and to report on the ethical issues associated with genetic screening. Its report, *Genetic Screening: ethical issues*[6], was published in 1993 and generated much public discussion. The scope of the Report goes beyond the interests of DH, and Ministers in a number of Government Departments will consider the reaction of public and professional interests before further action is decided upon.

(v)   Lifestyle and treatment

The activities of a small number of doctors who have used their professional position to offer patients diagnoses or advice based on spiritual or moral, rather than medical, grounds has given rise to new and clearer guidance from the General Medical Council (GMC). Although the expression of personal opinions or faith during a consultation is not itself considered improper, a doctor would be in breach of the Council's guidance where there was evidence that he or she had failed to provide an adequate standard of care. Doctors who cause patients distress by inappropriate or insensitive expression of personal views will be considered not to be providing the considerate care which patients are entitled to expect and which the GMC, as the regulatory body, requires. Guidance on this issue is expected to be released by the GMC during 1995.

References

1. Department of Health. *On the State of the Public Health: the annual report of the Chief Medical Officer of the Department of Health for the year 1991.* London: HMSO, 1992; 137-8.
2. Committee on the Ethics of Gene Therapy. *Report of the Committee on the Ethics of Gene Therapy.* London: HMSO, 1992 (Cm. 1788). Chair: Sir Cecil Clothier.

3.   Department of Health. *Appointment of Members of Gene Therapy Advisory Committee*. London: Department of Health, 1993 (Press Release: H93/1056).
4.   NHS Management Executive. *Monitoring Issues Outside Corporate Contracts: 1992/93*. Heywood (Lancashire): Department of Health, 1992 (Executive Letter (EL(92)66).
5.   Department of Health. *Services for Genetic Disorders*. Heywood (Lancashire): Department of Health, 1993 (Professional Letter PL/CMO(93)5, PL/CNO(93)4).
6.   Nuffield Council on Bioethics. *Genetic Screening: ethical issues: report of a working party*. London: Nuffield Council on Bioethics, 1993. Chair: Professor Dame June Lloyd.

(g)   London Implementation Group

Following publication of the report[1] of Sir Bernard Tomlinson's Inquiry into the organisation of health care and medical education and research in London, Ministers consulted widely before publishing the Government's response, *Making London Better*[2], in February. *Making London Better*[2] set out a strategic framework for London's health services with four main elements:

-   the development of higher quality, more accessible local community and primary health care services;

-   the provision of a better balanced hospital service, on fewer sites, to meet the needs of London's resident, working and visiting populations;

-   the rationalisation and development of specialist hospital services, to safeguard standards in patient care and medical education and research whilst securing value for money; *and*

-   the merging of free-standing undergraduate medical schools with multi-faculty colleges of the University of London for the benefit of medical teaching and research.

The London Implementation Group (LIG) was set up to take forward this major programme of work. A London Initiative Zone was established as a focus for new investment and new approaches in primary health care and community-based services, with an additional £40 million allocated in 1993/94 to support primary care development plans. Strategic plans for 1994-99 are being prepared by Family Health Services Authorities (FHSAs). £170 million will be made available over six years for community and primary health care capital projects, and £7.5 million over three years for voluntary sector schemes to reduce the need for hospitalisation or to enable early discharge.

The LIG has also established a mental health reference group to advise on a range of issues and challenges related to mental health services in London. Membership of this group is drawn from a wide range of health and local authority organisations, with emphasis on promoting the needs of mentally ill people when changes to primary and secondary health care are being considered. Independent reviews of six specialties (cancer, cardiac, neurosciences, plastics and burns, renal and children's services) were commissioned, and reported in June. The findings, alongside a review of research in Special Health Authorities, hospital site option appraisals, the views of health care commissioning agencies and authorities, and assessments of academic requirements, have helped LIG and the local Regional Health Authorities (RHAs) to develop proposals for the reconfiguration of the acute hospital service in London. Ministers announced the first wave of decisions on 15 December 1993[3]. Any proposed changes will be subject to normal statutory consultation procedures.

A clearing house has been set up to assist staff who may be displaced as a result of the changes brought about by *Making London Better*[2], and to help to minimise the loss of skills, knowledge and experience to the NHS. LIG is also working closely with the Higher Education Funding Council for England, to investigate ways to facilitate the merger of London medical schools.

References

1. Department of Health, Department for Education. *Report of the Inquiry into London's Health Service, Medical Education and Research: presented to the Secretaries of State for Health and Education by Sir Bernard Tomlinson.* London: HMSO, 1992.
2. Department of Health. *Making London Better.* Heywood (Lancashire): Department of Health, 1993.
3. Department of Health. *Virginia Bottomley announces progress on 'Making London Better'.* London: Department of Health (Press Release: H93/1127).

(h)   Research and development

(i)   *Report of the Advisory Council on Science and Technology*

The Government response to the report[1] on medical research and health of the Advisory Council on Science and Technology (ACOST) was co-ordinated by DH and published on 15 June[2]. The ACOST report made a number of proposals to improve the way in which advances in medical research are translated into better patient care. The success of the health care industry was recognised and a number of recommendations were made to build on its achievements.

The Government response welcomed the report, which shared common themes with *Research for Health*[3] and *Realising Our Potential*[4]. The response identified a key strategic role for Government in promoting alliances in health and medical research. Action taken in response to the ACOST report includes:

- support for the proposal to introduce a MEDLINK sub-programme within the existing LINK initiative;

- the establishment of programmes to implement and monitor the adoption and diffusion of clinical standards through the NHS research and development strategy;

- the development of the Standing Group on Health Technology Assessment to handle questions of safety and efficacy of surgical procedures; *and*

- the introduction of good clinical practice training programmes in the NHS, under the guidance of RDsRD.

(ii)   ***White Paper on science, engineering and technology***

The White Paper *Realising Our Potential: a strategy for science, engineering and technology*[4] was launched in May. It represented the first major policy review of science and technology for over 20 years and was intended to help the scientific, engineering and business communities to secure the maximum economic benefit from science and technology, whilst continuing to support excellence in basic research. A need for stronger links between industrial and Government strategies was highlighted in the White Paper, which placed special emphasis on wealth creation and the customer-contractor principle for Departmental research and development. It noted the contribution of advances in health technologies to the wealth-creating capacity of the nation through improved services and quality of life. New initiatives following from the White Paper include:

-   the creation of a new Council for Science and Technology which will provide outside independent and expert advice to Government;

-   the annual publication of a forward look at Government-funded science and technology research, which will provide industry and the research community with an up-to-date statement of Government strategy;

-   the Technology Foresight Programme, which aims to identify generic technologies which are expected to bring future social and economic benefits; *and*

-   a campaign to enhance public understanding of science.

(iii)   ***Research for health***

The report *Research for Health*[3], published in June, summarised progress and set the direction of DH's new research and development strategy, first announced in April 1991. It identified a dual challenge: to maximise the benefits of science and technology for health and health care, and to apply research rigour to the everyday problems encountered in the NHS and public health and social services. *Research for Health* embraces the NHS research and development programme, DH's Centrally Commissioned Programme (CCP) and the wider research and development strategy. The overall aim is to provide a coherent research-led approach to the challenges that the Department and the NHS will face in the 21st century.

In the NHS, the research and development strategy has been designed to establish a coherent infrastructure to support the promotion of health and the provision of health care. The aim is to change a service inclined to act as a passive recipient of new technologies into one with a strong research base that can critically review its own needs. The CCP aims to provide information derived from research so that it can be used for the development of policies related to the factors which affect public health, with special reference to the priorities of the

189

strategy for health[5] and the quality and efficacy of social care. A new Code of Practice was introduced during 1993 to specify DH's principles and practices for the commissioning and management of research and development. The main aims of the wider strategy are to develop alliances to take advantage of technical advances, to encourage the involvement of other participants in national research and development programmes, and to explore the possibilities of international links.

References

1. Cabinet Office, Advisory Council on Science and Technology. *A Report on Medical Research and Health.* London: HMSO, 1993.
2. Department of Health. *The Government's Response to the ACOST Report on Medical Research and Health.* London: Department of Health, 1993.
3. Department of Health. *Research for Health.* London: Department of Health, 1993.
4. Office of Publice Service and Science. *Realising Our Potential: a strategy for science, engineering and technology.* London: HMSO, 1993 (Cm. 2250).
5. Department of Health. *The Health of the Nation: a strategy for health in England.* London: HMSO, 1992 (Cm. 1986).

(i)   Dental health

(i)   *Dental health of the nation*

Dental epidemiological research in 1992/93 included work on the child dental health survey (the third of a ten-year series); the dental status, needs and demands of elderly people and, as part of the National Diet and Nutritional Survey, a study into the dental health of children aged 1.5 to 4.5 years. Results from all of these studies should be published during 1994. Early indications from the 1993 national survey of children's dental health, which involved some 17,000 children, indicate that the decline in caries in deciduous teeth has now levelled out in many areas: children living in some inner-city areas, and members of some ethnic minority groups, are still at increased risk. There are encouraging signs of lower rates of dental caries in children's permanent teeth, and of improved dental health and tooth retention in all adult age-groups. Nevertheless, a need remains for population preventive measures, such as water fluoridation and effective oral health education.

(ii)   *General dental services*

In July 1992, Sir Kenneth Bloomfield was appointed by the Secretary of State for Health to conduct a fundamental review of the remuneration system for general dental practitioners and to identify options for change. His report[1] was followed by a period of extensive consultation. In June, the House of Commons Health Select Committee published its report[2] into dental services. Both reports noted the lack of consensus about solutions among the dental profession, and this was confirmed during the consultation exercise.

The Bloomfield report analysed the existing remuneration system and concluded that it had worked well since its inception in the 1940s. Although introduction of the new dental contract in 1990 had not been the direct cause of difficulties experienced in 1992, it had introduced some uncertainty into the forecasting needed to operate the remuneration system. Sir Kenneth believed that the existing system could be modified and he identified possible ways to adapt it. However, he concluded that some important weaknesses would remain without more radical change.

Several recommendations were also made in the Health Committee report. Key points included the need for an oral health strategy for England and a stable system of remuneration to reward high-quality work and high productivity, but which could be effectively monitored. The Committee recommended that there should be greater co-ordination of local services and increased involvement by local health authorities in the delivery of primary dental care, and that dental treatments should be split into three categories: diagnostic and preventive services, maintenance services and advanced treatments. The Government welcomed the Committee's report in a response published in August[3], which contained the statements "the Government agrees that an oral health strategy is important. One will be published", and "the Government agrees that improving oral health is the aim of any system of dental remuneration; it is fully committed to developing a system that achieves this".

Since October 1990, when the new dental contract was introduced, patients have formally registered for continuing care with their dentist. At 31 December 1993, a total of 32,105,861 people were registered in Great Britain, of whom 24,813,222 were adults and 7,292,639 were children.

(iii)   Community dental services

The community dental services treatment statistics collection Form KC64 was revised during 1993 in response to advice given by NHS Trusts, DHAs and consultants in dental public health. After careful consideration, the introduction of the new version of the form was delayed to allow for a longer period for planning and consultation and to take into account any relevant changes that may arise from the fundamental review of the remuneration of general dental practitioners.

The third ten-year survey of dental caries among children in the UK was conducted in the first half of 1993. Over 17,000 children aged between 5 and 15 years had a dental examination at school by one of a team of 76 dentists seconded from the community dental service. 96% of the schools approached co-operated with the study, and 90% of the children selected at these schools were successfully examined: 559 primary schools and 139 secondary schools took part.

The proposals in *Managing the New NHS*[4], announced in October by the Secretary of State for Health, will have implications for the future programme of dental health surveys conducted by the British Association for the Study of Community Dentistry. The 1993/94 survey of 5-year-old children will go ahead with the co-operation of existing Regional co-ordinators and trainers but future surveys are likely to based on the new NHS management structure.

(iv)   Hospital dental services

The number of hospital dentists in England rose by 4.6% from 1,183 whole-time equivalent posts to 1,238 between September 1991 and September 1992. There were 443 consultants in post, an apparent increase of 10.8%, but the rise is due almost entirely to under-reporting in 1991. The number of senior registrars fell by 3% from 101 to 98 and the number of senior house officers rose by 10.6% from 227 to 251.

Compared with 1991/92, there was a rise in new outpatient referrals to consultant clinics in all four dental specialties in 1992/93: referrals rose by 3.9% from 379,496 to 394,268 in oral surgery; by 5.3% from 56,084 to 59,074 in restorative dentistry; by 12% from 24,719 to 27,685 in paediatric dentistry; and by 13.3% from 91,464 to 103,625 in orthodontics. Repeat attendances at outpatient clinics in 1992/93 rose by 0.9% from 721,457 to 727,773 in oral surgery; and by 1.4% from 649,049 to 657,968 in orthodontics. Repeat attendances fell by 8.1% from 369,411 to 339,363 in restorative dentistry and by 11.7% from 89,924 to 79,358 in paediatric dentistry.

(v)   Continuing education and training for dentists

By 1 October, all dentists applying for inclusion in FHSA lists of practitioners who have agreed to provide general dental services (GDS) had to have completed a year's vocational training in the GDS under an approved trainer unless they could satisfy the Dental Vocational Training Authority that they had acquired experience or training equivalent to such vocational training, or were in categories exempted from this requirement. Vocational training schemes for the GDS continued to expand and by December there were 410 trainees in 39 regionally based programmes.

As in previous years, the Committee for Continuing Education and Training identified several topics as priority areas for the training of general dental practitioners in 1993/94: 'hands-on' courses; the management of elderly or disabled patients and those with special needs; venepuncture; the training of trainers, examiners and advisers; research techniques; and courses to reinforce distance learning programmes. These courses are arranged by Regional postgraduate dental deans or directors of dental education, with funding provided by DH under the provisions of Section 63 of the Health Services and Public Health Act 1968[5].

During 1993, DH continued to produce and distribute distance learning material to general dental practices, including four training video tapes, computer-assisted learning programmes and further information related to the *Pathways in Practice* project, developed in collaboration with the Faculty of General Dental Practitioners of the Royal College of Surgeons of England.

(vi) Dental research

Dental needs of elderly people

The University of Newcastle-upon-Tyne was commissioned to study the dental health status, needs and demands of a sample of elderly people in England. Preliminary results indicate large geographical differences in the proportion of the population who are edentulous; 60% of the total sample considered they did not need to visit a dentist.

Dental capitation

The universities of Manchester and Birmingham were commissioned to investigate the dental health of children registered in the capitation scheme for the provision of care in the NHS by general dental practitioners.

Dental radiographs

The University of Manchester reported on a commissioned clinical study to evaluate a radiographic quality assurance programme. Film holders and simple monitoring devices have been recommended for routine use; parts of this study will be published during 1994.

References

1. Department of Health. *Fundamental Review of Dental Remuneration: report of Sir Kenneth Bloomfield KCB.* London: Department of Health, 1992.
2. House of Commons, Health Committee. *Dental Services: fourth report from the Health Committee: session 1992-93.* London: HMSO, 1993 (HC 264, vols I-II).
3. Department of Health. *Government Response to the Fourth Report from the Health Committee Session 1992-93: dental services.* London: HMSO, 1993 (Cm. 2308).
4. Department of Health. *Managing the New NHS.* Leeds: Department of Health, 1993.
5. *Health Services and Public Health Act 1968.* London: HMSO, 1968.

CHAPTER 10

INTERNATIONAL HEALTH

(a)   England, Europe and health

Many of the health challenges encountered in England and the United Kingdom (UK) as a whole are also found in the rest of Europe. Diseases have little respect for national boundaries. Ageing populations, technological advances and increased expectations lead to greater demands on any nation's health services, but the fact that these challenges are faced together is a source of great hope. The knowledge gained from dealing with health issues across the European Community (EC) will be of great benefit.

Nowhere can be insulated from the huge changes taking place in the world, and all industrialised countries share the challenge of rising health care costs and the need to combat preventable diseases. Political changes in central and eastern Europe have led to increased numbers of refugees and other migrants to the EC - groups that have distinct health needs and present new challenges to the public health systems of host countries.

(b)   The European Community

(i)   Treaty on European Union (Maastricht)

The Maastricht Treaty came into force on 1 November and the new public health article (Article 129) is beginning to influence the way that the EC approaches public health issues. Most notably, the European Commission has responded to pressure from the UK and other countries to improve the co-ordination between its activities and to provide more consistency between one Presidency and the next.

The Framework for Action in the Field of Public Health proposes Community actions, some of which continue existing work, in the fields of cancer; drug dependence; AIDS and other communicable diseases; health promotion and education; the exchange of health data; accidents; rare diseases; and pollution-related diseases. The Commission is also exploring mechanisms whereby the health consequences of other EC policies can be recognised and adapted to public health targets.

Member States remain responsible for the health of their citizens and the provision of health care services, and Community action takes place, in accordance with the principle of subsidiarity, only when it adds to what could be achieved by individual Member States alone, and is proportionate to the goal being sought.

(ii)   *European Economic Area*

The European Economic Area (EEA) will come into force on 1 January 1994, effectively extending the EC Single Market to five member countries of the European Free Trade Association (EFTA) - namely Austria, Finland, Iceland, Norway and Sweden, of which all but Iceland are also negotiating to become full members of the EC. These states will adopt almost all existing EC Single Market legislation and will take on new measures as they are adopted by the EC, with the opportunity to influence any new proposals. Provisions related to health issues include the mutual recognition of qualifications and the regulation of food safety and pharmaceuticals. There will also be closer co-operation between EC and EEA countries in a number of areas, such as research and development and the environment.

(iii)   *The Council of Health Ministers*

There were two meetings of the Council of Health Ministers during the year. The first was held on 27 May under the Presidency of Denmark. The main development was the adoption of a Resolution that set out guidelines for the Framework for Action in the Field of Public Health. The European Commission responded to some of these measures at the second Council of the year, held on 13 December under the Presidency of Belgium. This meeting also adopted Resolutions on the conduct of the 'Europe Against Cancer' and 'Europe Against AIDS' programmes, and agreed that the next European Drug Prevention Week should take place in October 1994 under the Presidency of Germany.

(iv)   *EC/WHO/Council of Europe*

Close co-operation between the EC, the World Health Organization (WHO) and the Council of Europe continued during 1993, with collaboration in a number of areas such as the EC's PHARE (Poland and Hungary Assistance for Economic Restructuring) and TACIS (Technical Assistance to the Commonwealth of Independent States) programmes, WHO's EUROHEALTH programme for Central and Eastern Europe, and a joint initiative to set up a network of health promoting schools in which the UK is an active participant. The WHO European Regional Committee meeting in September passed a Resolution to request its Regional Director to sustain efforts to ensure the continued success of rapprochement, and urged countries to support this initiative.

(v)   *Free movement of people*

Health professionals

The number of health professionals from other Member States working in the UK is small and most come for short periods to gain experience. In 1993, 1,145 doctors with qualifications from other Member States obtained full registration with the General Medical Council, 90 dentists with the General Dental Council, 18 pharmacists with the Royal Pharmaceutical Society of Great Britain, 438 nurses and 19 midwives with the UK Central Council for Nursing, Midwifery and Health Visiting, and 224 with the Council for the Professions Supplementary to Medicine (3 chiropodists, 23 dietitians, 41 occupational therapists, 139 physiotherapists and 18 radiographers).

Patients

EC Social Security Regulation 1408/71 continued to operate satisfactorily, co-ordinating health care cover for people moving between Member States. The main categories covered were temporary visitors, detached workers and pensioners transferring their residence to another Member State. In 1993, 540 applications by UK patients for referral to other Member States specifically for treatment of pre-existing conditions were approved by DH. About 320 citizens of other Member States were treated in the UK on the same basis.

(vi)   Draft Directive on Data Protection

During the year discussions continued on a draft EC Directive on Data Protection. If adopted as currently drafted, the Directive would have considerable implications for the processing of personal health information. UK law contains specific safeguards on the processing of computerised data and gives individuals the right of access to their own health records. The confidentiality of personal health information is protected by duties in common law and the ethical obligations of health professionals.

The UK's concerns about the impact of the Directive in the health sector have been conveyed to the European Commission and other Member States, and discussions will continue during 1994 in an Internal Market Council Working Party.

(vii)   Smoking

The Council of Health Ministers reached conclusions on the European Commission's interim report on smoking in public places at its May meeting. The conclusions encouraged the Commission to include an assessment of the efficacy of the measures taken by Member States in its next report. The Council also discussed draft conclusions on the importance of tobacco taxation in reducing smoking. The proposed EC Directive to ban tobacco advertising continued to be discussed by the Council, but without agreement.

(viii)   Elderly and disabled people

The 1993 'European Year of Older People and Solidarity Between Generations' was launched in the UK by the Secretary of State for Health on 17 December 1992. During 1994, the European Commission will evaluate this initiative's main achievements to inform future programmes.

The third EC Action Programme to assist disabled people, HELIOS II, was adopted by the Council of Health Ministers on 23 February. DH, working closely with other Government Departments, has selected 78 UK participants that represent examples of good practice in the areas of social and educational integration, and functional and employment rehabilitation.

(ix) AIDS and HIV infection

Support continued during 1993 for various projects under the 'Europe against AIDS' programme, the AIDS component of the Biomedicine and Health Research Programme and the AIDS assistance programme for developing countries.

International World AIDS Day is held each year on 1 December. Government and voluntary bodies sponsored a number of initiatives to increase the public's awareness of HIV and AIDS and their impact on individuals and society. The UK response, co-ordinated by the National AIDS Trust, centred on WHO's theme for 1993, 'The Time to Act'.

(x) Pharmaceuticals

The EC took further initiatives to harmonise the licensing and control of medicines throughout the Community, including the adoption of future medicines licensing arrangements. These Future Systems were negotiated for the UK by the Medicines Control Agency and are described on page 179. The proposed European Medicines Evaluation Agency (EMEA) will be based in London and should come into operation in January 1995 (see page 179).

In August, DH agreed a new Pharmaceutical Price Regulation Scheme with the British pharmaceutical industry: like its predecessor, the new scheme had to meet the requirements of the EC Directive 89/105/EEC on the transparency of measures regulating the pricing of medicinal products for human use. This Directive does not aim to set EC prices for medicinal products but to ensure the transparency of Member States' own systems to control prices.

DH was also involved in discussions on a draft European Commission communication on policy for the pharmaceutical industry in the EC. The first draft set out means to improve the competitiveness of the European pharmaceutical industry, and a final version should be published during 1994.

(xi) Research and information technology

EC research and development is co-ordinated within medium-term Framework Programmes; currently research is part of the Third Framework Programme (1990-94). Discussions continue to commission a fourth programme, which is likely to start in 1995, and which will be larger than previous programmes. Three areas in the Framework Programmes are of particular interest to DH: the Biomedical and Health Research Programme (BIOMED), which covers prevention, care and health systems, major health problems and diseases, the human genome and biomedical ethics (work on this project is in conjunction with the Medical Research Council [MRC]); the Advanced Informatics in Medicine Programme, which seeks to support a common approach to health care information and telecommunications; and the Radiation Protection Research Programme (part of the EURATOM programme).

(xii)   Food safety

The EC General Food Hygiene Directive, adopted in June, sets out general hygiene principles and conditions for foodstuffs to apply throughout the food chain after harvesting or slaughter. Following the adoption of a number of product-specific food hygiene Directives, all food businesses will be subject to Single Market hygiene measures.

For implementation in the UK, the Government plans to lay down Regulations in July 1994, and these should come into force the following year. The Directive will simplify domestic food hygiene legislation. Key provisions include an emphasis in the Directive on the need for food businesses themselves to identify and control risks, and for industry to develop voluntary guides to good hygiene practice in collaboration with enforcement agencies, consumers and the Government.

The Directive allows the European Commission to propose legislation on temperature controls for food. In late 1993, the UK Government consulted widely on proposals to simplify domestic and EC controls in the belief that the complexity of current regulations does not benefit the food industry or consumer safety.

Directive on Scientific Co-operation in the Examination of Questions Relating to Food

This Directive, which allows scientific bodies nominated by Member States to carry out food safety evaluations on behalf of the EC, came into effect in June. The UK is working closely with the Commission and other Member States to develop procedures to ensure effective implementation of the Directive.

(c)   Relations with Central and Eastern Europe

The Secretary of State for Health visited Russia and Kazakhstan in April, accompanied by 15 representatives of the UK health care industry. She had discussions with the Russian Health Minister and signed a new Health Co-operation Agreement in Moscow, and visited Yekaterinburg, in the Urals Region of Sverdlovsk, which is the main centre of activity in Russia of the British Health Care Consortium (a group of leading health care and pharmaceutical companies). National Health Service (NHS) Overseas Enterprises continued to provide expert planning advice and training in health care management to the Sverdlovsk regional government.

The Secretary of State for Health also visited Almaty in Kazakhstan where she met the President and the Health Minister, with whom she signed a joint Declaration on co-operation in health care. The British Health Care Consortium also signed a collaborative agreement with the Kazakhstan Ministry of Health, and Amersham International signed a protocol for a co-operative venture to establish vaccine production.

The Health Co-operation Agreement with Russia was added to the existing bilateral agreements with Bulgaria, the Czech and Slovak Republics, Hungary, Poland, and Romania, as well as the former Soviet Union. Exchanges with these countries included visits to the UK from Bulgaria to study pulmonary health and attend a pathology conference, and from Poland to study health care management and gastro-enterology. UK specialists visited Hungary to advise on autism in children, general practitioner training, and health service organisation and planning. Delegates from the UK attended conferences in Hungary on gerontology and the nursing input to the care of patients with AIDS, and on neonatology in Poland. In Romania, a multi-disciplinary team from Guy's Hospital organised a workshop on the planning and delivery of services for children with disabilities. Contacts between various UK and Russian institutes, universities and hospitals were maintained and new links were established.

The WHO European Office continued to assist the countries of Central and Eastern Europe under its EUROHEALTH Programme. The UK also played a full part in international efforts to assist victims of the conflict in the former Yugoslavia. However, it became apparent during 1993 that medical facilities, particularly in Bosnia, had declined to such an extent that it was no longer possible for some patients to receive essential medical treatment locally. In response to requests for international assistance, the UK agreed to accept a number of the sick and injured for treatment by the NHS.

These patients had first to be assessed by the Medical Committee of the United Nations High Commission for Refugees (UNHCR) and recommended for medical evacuation in view of the seriousness of their conditions. Urgent arrangements were then made, involving the International Organisation for Migration and several Government departments to ensure that the evacuees were brought to this country as quickly as possible. The Emergency Planning Co-ordination Unit in DH was responsible for making the necessary arrangements with the NHS.

The first patient to be treated by the NHS in 1993 was Irma Hadzimuratovic, a five-year-old child from Sarajevo, who was brought to Great Ormond Street Hospital, London, on 9 August. Thereafter, up to the end of the year, a further 36 patients (including seven children) were brought to the UK. The majority were cared for by hospitals in London, Birmingham and Leeds. As far as possible, the patients were treated near Bosnian refugee centres so that they could keep in close touch with any relatives who had joined them in the UK. These relatives are also entitled to medical care by the NHS, where necessary. At the end of the year the medical evacuation programme was still continuing.

(d) Council of Europe

DH officials served on the European Health Committee and the Steering Committee on Bioethics (see page 184). The UK participated in select committees and working groups on a range of health issues, including the education and training of nurses, nursing research, early intervention against HIV infection and equity and efficiency. Under the Partial Agreements in the health field, DH continued to be involved in work on the harmonisation of standards and the production of guidelines for the use of pesticides, colourings and food additives, detergents, cosmetics and medicines. The UK continued to participate in the production of the European Pharmacopoeia monographs: the 870 monographs published to date represent about 60% of the target of 1,500 published monographs by the year 2000.

The Committee of Ministers, on the advice of the European Health Committee, adopted Recommendations on medico-social aspects of child abuse, multi-professional education of health staff, health manpower planning and standards/guidelines for clinical trials of blood products. Recommendations on the role and training of community pharmacists and contaminants in food were adopted under the Partial Agreements in the health field.

UK experts continued to participate in the Council's initiatives to establish closer links between European transplantation centres, particularly in respect of the rapid exchange of information, reduction of waiting lists, training of transplant co-ordinators and viral risks in transplantation. The UK was closely involved in the Council of Europe's activities in blood transfusion, including quality assurance in transfusion services and emphasis of the principles of self-sufficiency and non-commercialisation.

The Council of Europe also organised activities on organisational aspects of health systems, training in health promotion and disease prevention, and ethical and legal issues in medicine and health care through its Demosthenes programme to assist the countries of Central and Eastern Europe.

(e) The Commonwealth

Commonwealth Health Ministers met in Geneva on 2 May, before the World Health Assembly. The UK delegation was led by the Chief Medical Officer and included the Chief Nursing Officer and the head of the Health and Population Division of the Overseas Development Administration. The meeting discussed the WHO Programme Budget, strategies on health and the environment, tuberculosis and AIDS, and the report of the Steering Group of the Commonwealth Health Development Programme (of which the UK is a member). The Chief Medical Officer also gave a report of the WHO Executive Board Working Group, which he chaired, on WHO's response to global change.

(f)   WHO

(i)   *European Regional Committee*

The WHO European Regional Committee met in Athens in September. The UK delegation was led by Dr Jeremy Metters, the Deputy Chief Medical Officer. Among items discussed were the report of the Interim Standing Committee of the European Regional Committee, European contributions to WHO's programme of work to the year 2001, the EUROHEALTH programme for Central and Eastern Europe and the Report of the Executive Board Working Group on the WHO Response to Global Change.

A Standing Committee of the European Regional Committee was established to succeed the Interim Standing Committee. Dr Metters was elected to serve on the new Committee, which will provide a closer link between the European Regional Committee and the Regional Office secretariat and represent the Regional Committee's views between annual meetings. Rules of procedure for the new Standing Committee and revised rules of procedure for the European Regional Committee were agreed.

The Regional Committee identified its priorities under the Ninth General Programme of Work, including the updating of the Region's 'Health for All in the year 2000' targets and promotion of the EUROHEALTH programme to assist the countries of Central and Eastern Europe. Members acknowledged the financial implications of the EUROHEALTH programme, given the state of health and health care services in many of the countries concerned, and urged the Regional Office to undertake only those tasks and projects for which it had available resources, and to co-operate with other countries and international organisations with an interest in the region. The Regional Director reported on progress to improve rapprochement between the European Regional Committee, the EC and the Council of Europe.

A Search Committee was appointed to identify the most suitably qualified candidates to contest the election for the post of Regional Director in 1995.

(ii)   *Executive Board*

In January, the Chief Medical Officer attended the 91st session of the WHO Executive Board in Geneva as the UK's nominated representative. Among the matters discussed were the Programme Budget for 1994-95; the election of the Director General of WHO; and the preliminary report of the Executive Board's Working Group on WHO's Response to Global Change, which had been set up under the chairmanship of the Chief Medical Officer to look at the future role of WHO and to recommend changes in its organisation.

Members of the Board expressed concern about proposed increases in the 1994-95 Programme Budget and the Director General was asked to submit a revised Budget to the World Health Assembly in May. After an election the Board recommended to the World Health Assembly that Dr Nakajima be re-elected as Director General for a further five-year term. The Chief Medical Officer introduced the preliminary report of the Working Group which he had chaired and undertook to report on priority areas which had emerged during the subsequent discussions to the Executive Board in May.

The Executive Board held its second meeting in May after the World Health Assembly. The concepts and principles of the Working Group report on WHO's Response to Global Change were endorsed and the Board asked its Programme Committee to examine the proposals put forward by the Director General to implement the report. Recommendations included changes in the method of election of the Director General and Regional Directors; the establishment of an administrative, budget and finance committee; the establishment of a committee to assist with the implementation of the suggested changes; and publication of an annual assessment of world health and WHO action. The proposed strategy was developed further at the Programme Committee meeting in November, attended by the Chief Medical Officer, and will be reviewed by the full Executive Board in January 1994.

(iii)   World Health Assembly

The UK delegation to the 46th World Health Assembly, held in Geneva in May, was led by the Chief Medical Officer. The delegation included the Chief Nursing Officer, the Ambassador and staff of the UK Mission in Geneva and the head of the Health and Population Division of the Overseas Development Administration.

The Chief Medical Officer delivered a speech to the plenary session of the Assembly on the theme of health development in a changing world, in which he drew attention to some of the major health problems facing the world today, such as malaria, tuberculosis and AIDS. On the recommendation of the Executive Board, Dr Nakajima was re-elected for a further five-year term as Director General.

The main item of discussion was the Programme Budget for the 1994-95 biennium. During the debate on individual programmes, delegates expressed satisfaction with continued improvement in the global control of poliomyelitis and passed a resolution urging Member States to reaffirm their commitment to its elimination. Concern was expressed, however, about the prevalence of malaria and tuberculosis and resolutions were passed to urge Member States to control these diseases. The Assembly also passed a resolution for the Director General to set up a study on the feasibility and practicability of a UN Programme on HIV/AIDS. The Assembly adopted 40 resolutions including one which sanctioned a Programme Budget of US$ 890 million for 1994-95. The UK will pay a contribution of US$19.7 million in each of these calendar years.

Table A.1: *Population age and sex structure, England, 1993, and changes by age, 1981-91, 1991-92, and 1992-93*

Age (in years)	Resident population at mid-1993 (thousands)			Percentage changes (persons)		
	Persons	Males	Females	1981-91	1991-92	1992-93
Under 1	633	325	309	10.9	-1.0	-3.6
1-4	2611	1338	1273	15.2	1.2	0.2
5-15	6668	3426	3242	-13.1	1.2	1.8
16-29	9859	5047	4813	4.7	-2.0	-2.5
30-44	10301	5196	5106	11.5	-0.1	0.8
45-64/59*	9560	5347	4212	-0.2	3.0	2.3
65/60-74**	5519	1951	3568	-3.2	0.3	0.7
75-84	2541	945	1597	17.6	-1.3	-2.7
85+	840	208	632	49.2	4.7	5.1
All ages	48533	23782	24751	3.0	0.4	0.3

* 45-64 years for males and 45-59 years for females.
** 65-74 years for males and 60-74 years for females.

Note: i. OPCS population estimates are now fully rebased to incorporate information from the 1991 Census.
ii. Figures may not add precisely to totals due to rounding.

Source: OPCS

Table A.2: *Five main causes of death at different ages (and percentages¹ of all causes of deaths), England, 1992*

Rank	All ages - 1 and over		1-14 years		15-34 years		35-54 years		55-74 years		75 years and over	
	Males	Females	Males	Females	Males	Females	Males	Females	Males	Females	Males	Females
1	Ischaemic heart disease	Ischaemic heart disease	Road vehicle accidents	Congenital anomalies	Road vehicle accidents	Road vehicle accidents	Ischaemic heart disease	MN* of bone, connective tissue, skin and breast	Ischaemic heart disease	Ischaemic heart disease	Ischaemic heart disease	Ischaemic heart disease
	29%	23%	18%	15%	21%	14%	28%	22%	34%	24%	27%	25%
2	Cerebro-vascular disease	Cerebro-vascular disease	Other causes of injury and poisoning†	Other causes of injury and poisoning†	Other causes of injury and poisoning†	Other causes of injury and poisoning†	MN* of digestive organs and peritoneum	MN* of genito-urinary organs	MN* of respiratory and intra-thoracic organs	MN* of digestive organs and peritoneum	Cerebro-vascular disease	Cerebro-vascular disease
	9%	15%	16%	15%	20%	12%	9%	10%	13%	10%	12%	17%
3	MN* of respiratory and intra-thoracic organs	MN* of digestive organs and peritoneum	Congenital anomalies	Diseases of the nervous system and sense organs	Suicide and self-inflicted injury	Suicide and self-inflicted injury	MN* of respiratory and intra-thoracic organs	MN* of digestive organs and peritoneum	MN* of digestive organs and peritoneum	Cerebro-vascular disease	Chronic obstructive pulmonary disease and allied conditions	Pneumonia
	9%	7%	11%	13%	17%	9%	8%	9%	10%	9%	8%	8%
4	MN* of digestive organs and peritoneum	Pneumonia	Diseases of the nervous system and sense organs	Road vehicle accidents	Diseases of the nervous system and sense organs	Diseases of the nervous system and sense organs	Other causes of injury and poisoning†	MN* of digestive organs and peritoneum	Cerebro-vascular disease	MN* of respiratory and intra-thoracic organs	MN* of respiratory and intra-thoracic organs	MN* of digestive organs and peritoneum
	8%	6%	11%	11%	5%	8%	6%	9%	7%	8%	7%	6%
5	Chronic obstructive pulmonary disease and allied conditions	MN* of bone, connective tissue, skin and breast	MN* of lymphatic and haema-topoietic tissue	MN* of lymphatic and haema-topoietic tissue	MN* of lymphatic and haema-topoietic tissue	MN* of bone, connective tissue, skin and breast	Suicide and self-inflicted injury	MN* of respiratory and intra-thoracic organs	Chronic obstructive pulmonary disease and allied conditions	MN* of bone, connective tissue, skin and breast	MN* of digestive organs and peritoneum	Mental disorders
	7%	5%	7%	5%	4%	7%	6%	7%	6%	8%	7%	4%
Remainder	38%	44%	36%	41%	33%	41%	43%	45%	30%	41%	39%	40%
All causes of death	251751	266646	996	726	5864	2579	17788	11243	102354	68888	124749	183210

¹ May not add up to 100 due to rounding. * MN = malignant neoplasm.

† 'Other causes of injury and poisoning' comprises categories of external injury and poisoning (E800-E999) excluding road vehicle accidents (E810-E829) and suicide (E950-E959).

Source: OPCS

Table A.3: *Relative mortality from various conditions when presented as numbers of deaths and future years of 'working life' lost, England and Wales, 1992*

Cause (ICD9 code)	Males Number of deaths (thousands) All ages	(%)	Males Years of 'working life' lost (thousands) Age 15-64	(%)	Females Number of deaths (thousands) All ages	(%)	Females Years of 'working life' lost (thousands) Age 15-64	(%)
All causes, all ages	272		915		287		544	
All causes, 28 days and over	270	(100)	832	(100)	285	(100)	480	(100)
All malignant neoplasms* (140-208)	75	(28)	183	(22)	64	(22)	195	(41)
Lung cancer (162)	23	(9)	39	(5)	10	(4)	20	(4)
Breast cancer+ (174)					13	(5)	59	(12)
Genito-urinary cancer (179-189)	14	(5)	16	(2)	9	(3)	35	(7)
Leukaemia (204-208)	2	(1)	14	(2)	2	(1)	16	(3)
Circulatory disease* (390-459)	122	(45)	201	(24)	124	(44)	74	(15)
Ischaemic heart disease (410-414)	79	(29)	144	(17)	67	(24)	32	(7)
Cerebrovascular disease (430-438)	25	(9)	26	(3)	39	(14)	23	(5)
Respiratory disease* (460-519)	30	(11)	36	(4)	31	(11)	21	(4)
Pneumonia (480-486)	9	(3)	14	(2)	16	(6)	6	(1)
Bronchitis, emphysema and asthma (490-493)	5	(2)	9	(1)	3	(1)	7	(1)
Sudden infant death syndrome (798.0)	0	(0)	15	(2)	0	(0)	8	(2)
All accidental deaths* (E800-E949)	6	(2)	131	(16)	4	(1)	39	(8)
Motor vehicle traffic accidents (E810-E819)	3	(1)	77	(9)	1	(0)	23	(5)
Suicide (E950-E959)	3	(1)	67	(8)	1	(0)	15	(3)

* These conditions are ranked as well as selected causes within these broader headings.   + Not calculated for male breast cancer.

Deaths under 28 days are excluded, except from 'All causes, all ages'.

Source: OPCS

Table A.4: *Trends in 'avoidable' deaths, England and Wales, 1979-92. Age-standardised mortality ratios (1979 = 100)*

Condition	SMR[1]												Actual number of deaths[4]	
	1979	1982	1983	1984	1985	1986	1987	1988	1989	1990	1991	1992	1979	1992
Hypertension/cerebrovascular (ages 35-64)	100	84	80	77	76	72	68	63	60	57	57*	55	9482	5181
Perinatal mortality[2]	100	77	71	69	67	65	61	60	57	55	55	51	9400	5213
Cervical cancer (ages 15-64)	100	90	90	91	91	97	89	84	80	77	73	68	1142	785
Hodgkin's disease (ages 5-64)	100	86	86	79	75	74	82	74	64	59	57*	59	365	229
Respiratory diseases (ages 1-14)	100	87	62	51	50	40	47	40	41	39	41	28	329	93
Surgical diseases[3] (ages 5-64)	100	77	71	78	66	72	53	69	52	58	55	60	262	155
Asthma (ages 5-44)	100	105	105	102	113	111	111	106	92	84	88	68	250	183
Tuberculosis (ages 5-64)	100	91	62	64	65	58	63	55	55	47	47	47	222	106
Chronic rheumatic heart disease (ages 5-44)	100	52	42	41	35	34	32	18	26	21	19	14	133	22
Total 'avoidable' deaths	100	81	76	74	72	70	66	62	59	57	57	54	21585	11967
All causes: ages 0-14 years	100	82	77	73	74	73	72	71	66	62	58	54	11132	6450
All causes: ages 15-64 years	100	92	90	88	88	86	84	82	80	78	76	74	127194	94491
All causes: all ages	100	94	93	89	92	89	86	85	85	82	82	84	591039	558313

[1] The standardised mortality ratio (SMR) for a condition is calculated by dividing the observed number of deaths by the expected number of deaths based on 1979 death rates.

[2] Stillbirths (2,929 in 1992) are included in perinatal mortality and total 'avoidable' deaths, but not in deaths from all causes.

[3] Appendicitis, abdominal hernia, cholelithiasis and cholecystitis.

[4] Excluding deaths of visitors to England and Wales.

* Revised from figure (58) quoted in 1991 Report.

Source: Calculated by Department of Health (SD2A) from data supplied by OPCS

206

Table A.5: *Live births, stillbirths, infant mortality and abortions, England[1], 1960-92*

Year	Live births Number	Stillbirths Number	Stillbirths Rate[2]	Early neonatal mortality (deaths under 1 week) Number	Early neonatal mortality (deaths under 1 week) Rate[3]	Perinatal mortality (stillbirths plus deaths under 1 week) Rate[2]	Post-neonatal mortality (deaths 4 weeks to under 1 year) Rate[3]	Infant mortality (deaths under 1 year) Rate[3]	Abortions[1] Rate[4]
1960	740859	14753	19.5	9772	13.2	32.5	6.3	21.6	-
1970	741999	9708	12.9	7864	10.6	23.4	5.9	18.2	87.6
1975	563900	5918	10.4	5154	9.1	19.4	5.0	15.7	149.9
1976	550393	5339	9.6	4468	8.1	17.6	4.6	14.2	148.7
1977	536953	5087	9.4	4070	7.6	16.9	4.5	13.7	152.7
1978	562589	4791	8.4	3975	7.1	15.4	4.4	13.1	157.7
1979	601316	4811	7.9	4028	6.7	14.6	4.5	12.8	158.8
1980	619371	4523	7.3	3793	6.1	13.4	4.4	12.0	164.5
1981	598163	3939	6.5	3105	5.2	11.7	4.3	10.9	168.8
1982	589711	3731	6.3	2939	5.0	11.2	4.5*	10.8	171.1
1983	593255	3412	5.7	2746	4.6	10.3	4.2	10.0	169.2
1984	600573	3425	5.7	2640	4.4	10.0	3.9	9.4	177.3
1985	619301	3426	5.5	2674	4.3	9.8	3.9	9.2	177.6
1986	623609	3337	5.3	2640	4.2	9.5	4.2	9.5	183.5
1987	643330	3224	5.0	2518	3.9	8.9	4.0	9.1	187.7
1988	654360	3188	4.8	2543	3.9	8.7	4.1	9.1	196.6
1989	649357	3056	4.7	2368	3.6	8.3	3.7	8.4	200.0
1990	666920	3068	4.6	2382	3.6	8.1	3.3	7.9	199.0
1991	660806	3072	4.6	2260	3.4	8.0	3.0	7.3	194.4
1992	651784	2777††	4.2†	2174	3.3	7.6†	2.3	6.5	190.1[5]

[1] Relates to England residents.   [2] Per 1,000 live births.   [3] Per 1,000 live and stillbirths.   [4] Per 1,000 conceptions (live births, stillbirths and abortions).   [5] Provisional.

* The post-neonatal mortality rate in 1982 has been incorrectly cited as 4.6 per 1,000 live births in recent Reports.

†† 1992 figures exclude 198 stillbirths of between 24 and 27 completed weeks gestation registered between 1 October 1992 and 31 December 1992, following the introduction of new legislation (see Chapter 1).

Source: OPCS

Table A.6: *Congenital malformations, England, 1980, 1985, 1992† and 1993†*

ICD Code(s)	Malformation	Live births*				Stillbirths**			
		1980	1985	1992	1993#	1980	1985	1992	1993#
	Malformed babies								
	Number	12704	12215	5637	5292	697	322	138	147
	Rate	205.4	197.2	86.5		11.2	5.2	2.1	
320-359.9, 740-742.9	**Central nervous system**								
	Number	1087	658	253	201	627	149	51	42
	Rate	17.6	10.6	3.9		10.1	2.4	0.8	
360-379.9, 743.0-743.9, 744.0-744.3	**Ear and eye**								
	Number	447	698	232	218	22	18	8	5
	Rate	7.2	11.3	3.6		0.4	0.3	0.1	
749.0-749.2	**Cleft lip/cleft palate**								
	Number	815	758	678	612	49	19	12	8
	Rate	13.2	12.2	10.4		0.8	0.3	0.2	
390-459.9, 745.0-747.9	**Cardiovascular**								
	Number	894	745	494	450	18	13	7	17
	Rate	14.5	12.0	7.6		0.3	0.2	0.1	
752.6	**Hypospadias/epispadias**								
	Number	930	1001	521	528	1	3	1	-
	Rate	15.0	16.2	8.0		0.0	0.0	0.0	
755.2-755.4	**Reduction deformities of limbs**								
	Number	292	329	178	213	21	7	4	9
	Rate	4.7	5.3	2.7		0.3	0.1	0.1	
754.5-754.7	**Talipes**								
	Number	2324	1879	738	612	43	19	4	7
	Rate	37.6	30.3	11.3		0.7	0.3	0.1	
758.0-758.9	**Chromosomal**								
	Number	523	520	468	372	16	16	16	22
	Rate	8.5	8.4	7.2		0.3	0.3	0.2	

† From January 1990 certain minor malformations are no longer notified, and have been excluded from the figures shown. For example, club foot of positional origin is now excluded from the category 'Talipes', ICD Codes 754.5-754.7. This change in notification practice largely accounts for the decrease in the number of malformations reported in some categories. The format of this table also differs from that in previous years to reflect ICD changes.

* Rates per 10,000 live births. ** Rates per 10,000 total births. # Provisional data; rates for 1993 are not available.

Source: OPCS

Table A.7: *Cancer* registrations by sex, age and site: males, England and Wales, 1989*

Numbers and percentages

	Age-group (years)															
	All ages	%	0-14 years	%	15-24 years	%	25-44 years	%	45-64 years	%	65-74 years	%	75-84 years	%	85 years and over	%
Eye, brain and other nervous system	2102	2	140	23	77	10	356	8	808	3	518	2	189	1	14	0
Mouth and pharynx	1932	2	6	1	16	2	149	3	780	3	565	2	332	1	84	1
Oesophagus	2957	3	0	0	2	0	65	1	898	3	1074	3	765	3	153	2
Lung	25276	25	2	0	8	1	327	7	6591	26	9769	29	7298	25	1281	20
Stomach	6608	7	1	0	2	0	116	3	1604	6	2313	7	2117	7	455	7
Pancreas	2930	3	2	0	0	0	72	2	733	3	1034	3	911	3	178	3
Large intestine and rectum	13492	13	1	0	10	1	369	8	3591	14	4523	13	4087	14	911	15
Prostate	12518	12	3	0	6	1	24	1	1478	6	4345	13	5304	18	1358	22
Bladder	8009	8	4	1	10	1	169	4	2090	8	2842	8	2339	8	555	9
Skin (melanoma)†	1354	1	6	1	32	4	305	7	534	2	273	1	171	1	33	1
Leukaemias and lymphomas	7901	8	293	47	320	40	888	20	2078	8	2117	6	1788	6	417	7
All other cancer	16163	16	159	26	316	40	1534	35	4654	18	4775	14	3896	13	829	13
Total cancer	101242	100	617	100	799	100	4374	100	25839	100	34148	100	29197	100	6268	100

* Cancer = malignant neoplasm.
† Melanoma of skin only (ICD9 code 172). Earlier reports included figures for other malignant neoplasm of skin (ICD9 code 173), which are greatly under-registered.

Note: Percentages may not add up to 100 due to rounding.

Source: OPCS

Table A.8: *Cancer* registrations by sex, age and site: females, England and Wales, 1989*

Numbers and percentages

Age-group (years)

	All ages	%	0-14 years	%	15-24 years	%	25-44 years	%	45-64 years	%	65-74 years	%	75-84 years	%	85 years and over	%
Eye, brain and other nervous system	1699	2	122	24	57	9	271	3	561	2	418	2	219	1	51	0
Mouth and pharynx	1162	1	7	1	5	1	85	1	328	1	346	1	281	1	110	1
Oesophagus	2224	2	0	0	0	0	23	0	420	1	610	2	816	3	355	3
Breast	27768	27	5	1	27	4	3459	41	11086	37	6279	23	4900	18	2012	19
Lung	11533	11	2	0	5	1	201	2	3138	10	4238	15	3186	12	763	7
Stomach	4211	4	0	0	2	0	66	1	550	2	1095	4	1671	6	827	8
Pancreas	3268	3	1	0	1	0	49	1	638	2	928	3	1171	4	480	4
Large intestine and rectum	13667	13	0	0	8	1	288	3	2720	9	3691	13	4742	18	2218	21
Ovary	5100	5	15	3	49	8	453	5	1973	7	1353	5	948	4	309	3
Cervix	4147	4	0	0	47	8	1465	17	1264	4	819	3	417	2	135	1
Other uterus	4073	4	0	0	4	1	179	2	1642	5	1130	4	834	3	284	3
Bladder	3344	3	2	0	6	1	82	1	690	2	1017	4	1071	4	476	4
Skin (melanoma)†	2249	2	6	1	71	12	569	7	765	3	420	2	314	1	104	1
Leukaemias and lymphomas	6946	7	206	40	214	35	550	7	1509	5	1756	6	1945	7	766	7
All other cancer	13101	13	146	29	115	19	676	8	2783	9	3520	13	4064	15	1797	17
Total cancer	104492	100	512	100	611	100	8416	100	30067	100	27620	100	26579	100	10687	100

* Cancer = malignant neoplasm.

† Melanoma of skin only (ICD9 code 172). Earlier reports included figures for other malignant neoplasm of skin (ICD9 code 173), which are greatly under-registered.

Note: Percentages may not add up to 100 due to rounding.

Source: OPCS

Table A.9: *Percentage of children immunised by their 2ⁿᵈ birthday and of children given BCG vaccine by their 14ᵗʰ birthday, England, 1980-92/93*

Year	Diphtheria	Tetanus	Polio	Whooping cough	Measles	Mumps/ rubella	BCG[1]
1980[2]	81	81	81	41	53	-	82
1981[2]	83	83	82	46	55	-	78
1982[2]	84	84	84	53	58	-	75
1983[2]	84	84	84	59	60	-	76
1984[2]	84	84	84	65	63	-	71
1985[2]	85	85	85	65	68	-	77
1986[2]	85	85	85	67	71	-	76
1987/88[2]	87	87	87	73	76	-	76
1988/89	87	87	87	75	80	7	71
1989/90	89	89	89	78	84	68	36[3]
1990/91	92	92	92	84	87	86	90[3]
1991/92	93	93	93	88	90	90	86[3]
1992/93	95	95	95	92	92	92	74

[1] Estimated percentage.
[2] Estimated percentage immunised by the end of the second year after birth.
[3] The school BCG programme was suspended in 1989 because there were insufficient supplies of BCG vaccine; figures for the subsequent two years were relatively higher as a result.

Sources: 1980-87/88: Form SBL 607
1988/89 onwards: Form KC51 (except BCG); KC50 (BCG)

Table A.10: *Cumulative totals of AIDS cases by exposure category, England, to 31 December 1993*

(Numbers subject to revision as further data are received or duplicates identified)

How persons probably acquired the virus	Number of cases			
	Male	Female	Total	%+
Sexual intercourse:				
between men	6010	-	6010	76
between men and women				
'High risk' partner*	25	62	87	1
Other partner abroad**	417	278	695	9
Other partner UK	42	32	74	1
Not known	4	2	6	<1
Injecting drug use (IDU)	187	85	272	3
IDU and sexual intercourse				
between men	127	-	127	2
Blood				
Blood factor	342	5	347	4
(eg haemophiliacs)				
Blood or tissue transfer				
(eg transfusion)				
Abroad	10	38	48	1
UK	17	18	35	<1
Mother to child	45	46	91	1
Other/undetermined	80	18	98	1
Total	7306	584	7890	100

* Includes men and women who had sex with injecting drug users, or with those infected through blood factor treatment or blood transfusion, and women who had sex with bisexual men.

** Includes persons without other identified risks who are from, or who have lived in, countries where the major route of HIV-1 transmission is through sexual intercourse between men and women.

+ Total does not add up to 100 because of rounding.

Source: CDSC

Figure A1: *Weekly deaths, England and Wales, 1992 and 1993, and expected deaths, 1993*

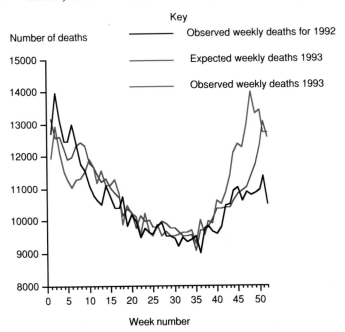

Key

Number of deaths

———— Observed weekly deaths for 1992

———— Expected weekly deaths 1993

———— Observed weekly deaths 1993

Week number

Notes: i. Deaths for the following weeks have been averaged to take account of the Easter and Christmas holidays: weeks 1991/52 and 1992/1; weeks 1992/16 and 17; weeks 1992/51, 52, 53 and 1993/1; and weeks 1993/14 and 15.

ii. Data are for 1-year-olds and over.

Source: OPCS

Printed in the UK for HMSO
Dd. 0299960. C30 13110